DR. ART ULENE'S
COMPLETE GUIDE TO
VITAMINS
MINERALS
AND
HERBS

DR. ART ULENE'S
COMPLETE GUIDE TO
VITAMINS
MINERALS
AND
HERBS

ART ULENE, MD

AVERY

a member of PENGUIN PUTNAM INC.   *New York*

Most Avery books are available at special quantity discounts for bulk purchase for sales promotions, premiums, fund-raising, and educational needs. Special books or book excerpts also can be created to fit specific needs. For details, write Putnam Special Markets, 375 Hudson Street, New York, NY 10014.

Avery
a member of
Penguin Putnam Inc.
375 Hudson Street
New York, NY 10014
www.penguinputnam.com

An application to register this book for cataloging has been submitted to the Library of Congress.

ISBN 0-58333-004-6

Printed in the United States of America

10 9 8 7 6 5 4 3 2 1

This book is printed on acid-free paper. ∞

Cover Designers: Oscar Maldonado and Doug Brooks
Editor: Peggy Hahn
Typesetter: Gary A. Rosenberg

Contents

Acknowledgments

The successful completion of this book required the hard work and dedication of many colleagues and friends. I would like to thank Jeffrey Blumberg, PhD, FACN, Professor of Nutrition at Tufts University; Kim Jordan, RD; Donald J. Brown, ND; and Valerie Ulene, MD for their valuable input from the scientific and nutritional perspectives. I am also grateful to Richard Trubo for his skillful writing and tireless work on this project; Kukla Vera for her guidance, talent, and tenacity; and Jamie McDowell for her competent administrative support.

A Message From Dr. Art Ulene

I was wrong about vitamins.

Twenty years ago, I told my television viewers that most people didn't need vitamin supplements. If you were eating well, I said, buying and consuming vitamin pills was a waste of money.

I certainly wasn't alone in this belief. At the time, few people in the medical community supported vitamin supplementation. Even today, most physicians, and many registered dietitians and nutritionists, insist that people in the United States get all the nutrients they need from diet alone. It's not surprising that health professionals feel this way. After all, that's what we were taught in school. That doesn't make it right, however.

Many years ago, a wise professor told me, "Fifty percent of what you'll learn in medical school will later be proven wrong." (I would have been spared a lot of anguish if he had told me *which* 50 percent.) Now I know that many of the pronouncements I heard about the uselessness of vitamin supplements simply aren't true. No matter what your age, no matter what your health status, new research shows that optimal doses of vitamins and minerals can improve the state of your health and greatly reduce your chances of developing many diseases and disorders once considered to be almost unavoidable.

For years, I preached a different sermon. With the best of intentions, I gave advice I would not offer today. So, what has changed my thinking? The answer is simple: Evidence from scientific studies supports the need for many vitamin and mineral supplements. This new knowledge requires all health-care professionals to reconsider our attitudes and amend the advice we have traditionally given about supplements. It has pointed me in a dramatically different direction, moving me to advocate a vitamin and mineral supplementation program for virtually everyone.

My beliefs about herbal remedies have changed as well. Herbs have been used for thousands of years to promote good health and treat minor physical problems. In fact, many of today's most popular mainstream medications are derived from plants. Nevertheless, there has been a scarcity of credible research supporting the use of most herbal remedies—until recently.

Thanks to a growing body of scientific evidence, I have come to believe that, in certain situations, herbal therapies can complement and, in some instances, provide alternatives to, traditional medications and conventional medical treatments. Unlike vitamins and minerals, herbs are not essential to life itself. But, in many cases, they can play an important role in promoting and sustaining good health. Research conducted at prestigious medical centers and published in major medical journals, including *JAMA (The Journal of the American Medical Association)* and the *Annals of Internal Medicine,* has demonstrated that some herbs can play a significant role in managing medical conditions ranging from high cholesterol and migraine headaches to memory problems and depression.

This book will present you with the evidence that has compelled me to change my mind about vitamin and mineral supplements and herbal remedies—and that may change your way of thinking, too. Many nutritional studies have reached some rather remarkable conclusions about optimal vitamin intakes and have proven—at least for some nutrients—that food alone will not provide these amounts, no matter how well you eat. Within these pages, you'll find general information that everyone should know about vitamins, minerals, and herbs, plus important strategies that will help you create a personalized nutrition program appropriate for your unique needs.

Of course, our knowledge is not yet complete. Although it's clear that some vitamins, minerals, and phytochemicals (plant chemicals) may offer protection against certain types of cancer, no one is certain how this occurs, or precisely how much of each of these cancer-fighting nutrients provides this protection. Some of these nutrients may enhance immune system function, but the ideal combinations and doses necessary to boost immunity have not been established. Many herbs may also produce health benefits, but in some instances, more studies of long-term use are needed to document the extent of the benefits or to prove their safety.

The evolving and growing body of research has led to a shift in the paradigm regarding vitamins, minerals, herbs, and other nutritional supplements. Many health-care professionals have changed their thinking about who needs supplements and how much they need. For example, research shows that we can no longer rely solely on diet to meet our vitamin and mineral requirements. In some cases (vitamin E, for example), you clearly *cannot* get the optimal amount of a vitamin from dietary sources alone. It has become apparent that it's difficult or impossible to get the optimal amounts of some nutrients from dietary sources alone. And government surveys show that most people don't even take in enough of the nutrients that they *should* be able to obtain through diet alone. In today's hectic world, when so many of us eat meals on the run, it's difficult to find time to prepare and eat the well-balanced, varied diets that are so important for good health.

It's important to keep in mind, however, that nutrient *supplements* are not nutrient *substitutes,* and should be used to complement a good diet, not to compensate for a poor one. Just because you take supplements, don't be tempted to dismiss or disregard health-promoting measures like reducing the fat in your diet, increasing your fiber intake, or quitting cigarette smoking. Instead, use vitamin and mineral supplements to complement a healthy lifestyle, and to ensure that you are getting optimal doses of the nutrients that are so critical to good health.

The purpose of this book is to help you achieve optimal health through nutrition. I hope that reading it inspires you to take a closer look at your own nutritional patterns, and to make whatever changes are necessary to achieve that goal. That's a big step toward optimal health and well-being.

—Art Ulene, MD

DR. ART ULENE'S
COMPLETE GUIDE TO
VITAMINS
MINERALS
AND
HERBS

Introduction

We live in an age of medical miracles. Procedures like bone marrow transplants and coronary bypass surgery are now being used to save lives that would have been lost a generation ago. These kinds of headline-grabbing technological breakthroughs are revolutionizing the way medicine is practiced today.

At the same time, a gentler—but no less important—revolution is taking place in the field of nutrition. As we learn more about the multitude of important functions that vitamins, minerals, and herbs perform in the body, our attitude toward them is changing.

Until recently, medical and nutritional experts recommended doses of each vitamin and mineral at a level just high enough to ward off deficiency diseases. Consume enough vitamin C, we were told, to prevent scurvy. Take just enough iron and folic acid, we were advised, to prevent anemia. And so on for each nutrient: vitamin A to prevent night blindness, vitamin D to prevent rickets, thiamin to prevent beriberi.

But new studies prove that some vitamins and minerals can do much more than protect us against deficiency disorders—especially when taken in optimal amounts. Evidence indicates that higher levels of selected nutrients may actually slow or prevent the aging-related physical deterioration that was once considered to be inevitable. Indeed, recent research suggests that optimal intake of certain vitamins and minerals may help many people prevent some of the most common chronic diseases and illnesses associated with aging, from cataracts to heart disease to cancer.

Today, many physicians believe we can significantly slow the aging process by changing the way we eat, increasing our physical activity levels, avoiding cigarettes, limiting alcohol intake, and taking supplements of certain vitamins, minerals, and herbs. This approach is part of an entirely new way of looking at aging and health. The goal of this approach is not merely to prevent disease, but to attain optimal health, or high-level wellness. Instead of spending our early years in good health and our later years in physical decline, we'll be able to live out our entire lives in excellent health.

I believe that the program presented in this book can help you achieve lifelong wellness. Will herbal remedies or vitamin and mineral supplements alone enable you to accomplish this goal? No. But there is now good reason to believe that, in combination with a healthy lifestyle, they can make a substantial contribution to your good health and longevity.

Despite mounting evidence about the importance of vitamins and minerals, however, most people in the United States still know little about these nutrients. Even with all the information about nutrition now available in magazines and newspapers and on television, radio, and the Internet, few people are familiar with the Recommended Dietary Allowances (RDAs) and Daily Values (DVs) for vitamins and minerals. And many lack the practical knowledge required to meet their nutritional needs. According to one survey, many people know that oranges are a good source of vitamin C, but can't say how many oranges it takes to meet their minimum needs. Nor can they describe the kinds and quantities of other foods that could supply this vitamin—or any other.

In a recent survey, about 38 percent of the people questioned stated that they took vitamin and mineral supplements on a daily or near-daily basis. About one-third of Americans said they have used herbs as well, though far fewer people use them regularly. The majority of these people recognized that they were not eating well-balanced diets, and admitted to taking supplements as "cheap insurance" against nutritional deficiencies. Some believed that the extra nutrients could enhance their levels of health and wellness. Some took vitamins, minerals, or herbs in the belief these supplements would help them sleep or accelerate their recovery from a cold.

In my own informal survey of supplement users, I found a small (but rapidly growing) group of people who took nutritional supplements because their doctors had recommended that they do so. Most of these people had been advised to take a multivitamin and mineral preparation that contained no more than the RDA for any particular nutrient.

When I asked regular supplement users how they decided which specific vitamins and minerals to take—and in what quantities—most said they guessed which preparations and doses would be best for them or selected brands they learned about through advertising. Others took the advice of store clerks or friends or relied on magazine articles. A few followed the recommendations of their doctors or pharmacists. Most of these people complained of confusion over the many nutritional products available in stores today.

What about the majority of people in the United States, who do not regularly take nutritional supplements? When interviewed, some said they took an occasional dose of one or more vitamins or minerals. But most said they did not supplement with vitamins and minerals because they believed they could get all of the nutrients they needed from the food they ate. And some indicated that they *would* use nutritional supplements if their doctors told them it was important to do so, but that hadn't happened yet.

Several major governmental agencies and professional organizations have finally acknowledged that most Americans simply aren't getting all of the critical nutrients they need from food alone. For example, only one-third of American women of childbearing age consume the level of folic acid (400 micrograms) deemed necessary to reduce the risk of neural tube birth defects. This is occurring in spite of the fact that the National Academy of Sciences, the U.S. Public Health Service, the American College of Obstetricians and Gynecologists, the American Academy of Pediatrics, the March of Dimes Foundation, and the Spina Bifida Society all recommend supplementation with 400 micrograms daily of folic acid for *all women of childbearing age,* no matter how well they eat, and whether or not they are pregnant or planning to get pregnant. To prevent birth defects, the supplementation must begin *before* pregnancy; half of all pregnancies in the United States are unplanned.

In addition to these statistics, other studies have shown that the average American woman consumes only about half of the recommended amount of calcium, which puts her at greater risk of developing osteoporosis, the bone-thinning disease. Both the National Osteoporosis Foundation and a National Institutes of Health Consensus Conference now agree that women should consume up to 1,500 milligrams of calcium daily—far more than the overwhelming majority of women are getting from the food they are eating.

Surprisingly, the diets of most people in this country do not include even the minimum amounts of vitamins and minerals recommended to avoid deficiency problems. Although the United States is the richest nation on earth, with healthful foods widely available in supermarkets nationwide, government surveys show that most people here do not consume the Recommended Dietary Allowances for many nutrients. Even fewer meet the Optimal Daily Allowance (ODA)—the dose I believe necessary to achieve optimal health. If "you are what you eat," it's no wonder that our doctors' offices and hospitals are filled with people whose illnesses might have been prevented or forestalled with better nutrition.

Be aware, however, that as important as it is to increase your intake of some nutrients, consuming excessive amounts of others—for example, preformed vitamin A, vitamin B_6, and iron—can cause serious toxic side effects and may even result in permanent physical damage. So, it's important to be prudent about your use of vitamin and mineral supplements to maximize the benefits while minimizing the risks.

This book is divided into four parts. Part One gives a broad background on vitamins, minerals, and herbs, describes what they can do for you, and provides guidelines to help you develop your personalized supplement program. Parts Two and Three provide an in-depth look at thirteen important vitamins and five essential minerals. You'll learn about the vital functions these nutrients perform in the body, and how to recognize the symptoms of deficiency or toxicity that may occur if you take in too little or too much of these vitamins and minerals. Optimal Daily Allowances for each nutrient are included in the individual chapters. Finally, Part Four provides an evaluation of many herbal remedies that are now available, along with information that will help you determine which herbs may be appropriate for your needs, and in what amounts you should take them.

The bottom line? It's time to question the old conventional wisdom about vitamin, mineral, and herbal supplements. Optimal health is more than just absence of disease—it's a state of exuberant wellness and of efficient, effortless function. If optimal health is your goal, this book will help you reach it.

Part One

The Basics

Chapter 1

The Facts About Vitamins and Minerals

There's no doubt that vitamins and minerals are important to good health. Researchers are continuing to learn more about how these nutrients work in the body in ways that may help enhance immunity, prevent degenerative disease, and slow aging. As a result, more people have become aware of the need to take in the optimal amounts of vitamins and minerals daily through diet, perhaps coupled with a good multinutrient supplement. Nevertheless, many people don't have a clear understanding of the vital functions that vitamins and minerals perform in the body.

Do you know the difference between fat-soluble and water-soluble vitamins, or how macro minerals differ from micro minerals? When you're in the supermarket, are you confident that you're choosing nutrient-packed foods, or do you think your diet may be lacking some of the vitamins and minerals you need to keep your body performing at its best? And if you do decide to take supplement pills, how do you know you're getting optimal levels of the nutrients you need to help ensure good health? This chapter will answer these questions—and more—by explaining the nature of vitamins and minerals, why they're so crucial for good health, and how to choose and use supplements.

VITAMIN BASICS

Vitamins are organic (carbon-containing) substances derived from plants and animals. They are called *micronutrients* because they are needed in relatively small amounts in the body when compared with the *macronutrients*—carbohydrates, fats, and proteins—that make up most of the diet and supply the body with energy. Micronutrients are not considered a source of energy, although some vitamins help convert calorie-containing nutrients into usable forms of energy. Both micronutrients and macronutrients are necessary for normal body growth, maintenance, and tissue repair.

Our knowledge about vitamins is relatively recent. Scientists identified the first vitamin—now known as vitamin A—in 1913. When researchers discovered that the chemical structure of this nutrient contained an amine (a nitrogen-containing chemical compound), they labeled the important substance *vitamine*—an amine vital to life. The "e" was eventually dropped from the name, and these nutrients have since been referred to as vitamins.

Vitamins can function as coenzymes in the body—that is, they "help" the enzymes that promote all of the body's biochemical processes. Enzymes are at the foundation of critical functions, including nerve transmission, muscle contraction, blood formation, protein metabolism, and energy production. Additionally, vitamins are necessary for the normal functioning of every organ in the body and are essential for sharp vision, normal blood clotting, and the formation of hormones and genetic material. Clearly, life itself would be impossible without these micronutrients!

Generally speaking, our bodies cannot manufacture vitamins, so we must obtain most of these nutrients from the foods we eat or from vitamin supplements. There are a couple of exceptions, however. Our skin manufactures vitamin D upon exposure to sunlight. In addition to vitamin D, our bodies can produce niacin—though somewhat inefficiently—if enough of the amino acid tryptophan is consumed.

All vitamins are either fat-soluble or water-soluble. Vitamins A, D, E, and K are fat-soluble vitamins. As their name suggests, these vitamins dissolve in liquid fats; they do not dissolve in water. The body absorbs fat-soluble vitamins through the intestinal tract membranes with the assistance of dietary fats and bile acids, which are substances produced by the liver that facilitate digestion. Once absorbed, these vitamins are transported and stored in the body's tissues, and in many cases the body can call upon these reserves if vitamin intake is low. Because these nutrients are stored in the body, toxic levels of vitamin A, D, and K in particular can accumulate relatively quickly when they are consumed consistently in high amounts.

The water-soluble vitamins include vitamin C and the B-complex vitamins. Vitamin B complex is actually a team of B vitamins, including B_1 (thiamin), B_2 (riboflavin), B_3 (niacin), B_5 (pantothenic acid), B_6 (pyridoxine), B_{12} (cobalamin), biotin, and folic acid. The body absorbs vitamin C and the B vitamins through the gastrointestinal tract without the help of dietary fats and bile acids. Unlike the fat-soluble vitamins, excess quantities of the water-soluble vitamins are excreted through urination or perspiration, so they are far less likely to accumulate to toxic levels in the body. However, this also means that we need to be more conscientious about consuming adequate amounts of water-soluble vitamins on a regular basis. These nutrients also tend to be less sturdy than fat-soluble nutrients and are more likely to be destroyed in storage, through cooking, or when exposed to light.

MINERAL BASICS

Although vitamins have traditionally received more attention, minerals are every bit as important. Whereas vitamins are organic substances, minerals are inorganic substances, meaning that they are not bound to carbon. Minerals originate in soil and water, and they are absorbed by the plants or eaten by the animals that make up the human diet.

Like vitamins, minerals are micronutrients that are needed in the body only in small amounts, although the body needs much larger quantities of many minerals than it requires of vitamins. Minerals can function as coenzymes, working with enzymes to activate the body's biochemical processes. They also help build strong bones and teeth and are necessary for the manufacture of hemoglobin, the oxygen-carrying component of the blood.

Minerals can be separated into two categories: *macro* minerals and *micro* minerals. Macro minerals are needed by the body in larger amounts than are micro minerals. The macro minerals—also known as *major* minerals—include calcium, chloride, magnesium, phosphorus, potassium, sodium, and sulfur. The micro minerals—often referred to as *trace* minerals—include chromium, copper, fluoride, iodine, iron, manganese, molybdenum, selenium, and zinc. Relatively little is known about some of the trace minerals, such as nickel and tin, but researchers believe that these nutrients are probably necessary in very small amounts.

Some minerals are also known as *electrolytes.* These are mineral salts that conduct the electrical energy needed to keep the body functioning. They are also responsible for muscle contraction and nerve impulse transmission. Chloride, sodium, magnesium, and potassium are electrolytes.

REDEFINING RECOMMENDED ALLOWANCES

The amounts of vitamins and minerals you need depend on the way you define your need. Are you taking nutrients to prevent deficiency symptoms? Or are you seeking to maximize your health? The recommended allowances established by the government are adequate to ensure that you will not experience nutrient deficiencies. However, for many vitamins and minerals, consuming the government's Recommended Dietary Allowances (RDAs) may not be enough to help you achieve the highest level of well-being. You may need to take in higher levels of some nutrients than the RDAs suggest to prevent chronic diseases and promote truly optimal health.

So what are the Recommended Dietary Allowances? The RDAs were first issued in the 1940s by the Food and Nutrition Board of the National Academy of Science's National Research Council. The Board periodically updates the RDAs, as continuing research reveals new findings on vitamins and minerals. Never intended as hard-and-fast requirements, the RDAs were created by nutritional scientists who calculated the body's need for each nutrient and then added a little more as a safety factor to compensate for individual variability. Not everyone is content with the RDAs, however. Many nutritional experts now believe that the recommended doses are not high enough to prevent chronic diseases and to promote optimal health.

The RDAs are somewhat complex because they include separate recommendations for each sex, for different age categories (from infancy to old age), and for pregnant or breast-feeding women. In the 1970s, officials of the U.S. Food and Drug Administration (FDA) decided to make the RDAs simpler and more accessible, particularly for placing this information on food-packaging labels. As a result, the FDA issued its own U.S. Recommended Daily Allowances, or USRDAs—a single recommendation for each vitamin and mineral. In general, USRDAs correspond to the highest RDA for each nutrient. More recently, the USRDAs were replaced with the Reference Daily Intakes, or RDIs, which are

Reading Food Labels

One of the best ways to ensure that your diet is rich in vitamins and minerals is to purchase foods that contain high amounts of these nutrients. These days, nutritional information is printed on food labels to help health-conscious shoppers select nutrient-rich foods. Millions of people in the United States—85 percent, according to one survey—already read food labels. Many depend on the information they get from these labels when they choose the items they will place in their supermarket carts; 75 percent of consumers say they pass up products if they don't like what they read.

Despite this apparent concern for good nutrition, however, many people find the nutritional information on food labels to be confusing and difficult to apply to their own diets in a useful way. While the FDA mandates that nearly all processed foods carry nutritional information, deciphering and utilizing that information has been a challenge. Fortunately, this seems to be changing. Since May 1994, the FDA has taken some of the guesswork out of the process, thanks to its new and more accessible labeling guidelines. The list of nutrients required on many food items is now considered more complete although, ironically, the new regulations do not require listing a few vitamins—thiamin, riboflavin, and niacin—because deficiencies of these nutrients are no longer considered a significant public health problem in the United States.

The most recent labeling system introduces new recommendations known as the Daily Values (DVs). These numbers provide information on specific food components—fat, saturated fat, cholesterol, sodium, total carbohydrate, fiber, potassium, protein, and some vitamins and minerals—that have been linked with the development of, or a decrease in, various chronic diseases.

also recommendations based on an average need. RDIs have been assigned to twenty-seven vitamins and minerals, and are represented on the new nutrition labels as percent Daily Values. (See "Reading Food Labels," on page 13.)

To further complicate labeling issues, in 1997 the National Academy of Sciences began reviewing its recommendations and compiling a new set of values to take the place of the RDAs. These Dietary Reference Intakes (DRIs) represent the Academy's recommendations for adequate nutrient intakes based on age, sex, and certain medical conditions. To date, the Academy has issued DRIs for some nutrients, including vitamin D, calcium, and magnesium.

WHAT YOU NEED TO KNOW ABOUT SUPPLEMENTS

As you read this book, you may decide that you want to consume more vitamins and minerals than you get from your meals—but you may need some pointers to help you choose and use your supplement products wisely. Below you will find some ideas to keep in mind when you make the trip to your local pharmacy or health food store.

Buying Supplements

It's easy to feel lost when you're confronted with rows upon rows of supplement products, but there's no need to panic! The following guidelines can help you navigate through the maze of vitamin and mineral choices.

Natural Versus Synthetic Supplements

Supplements can be divided into two categories: natural and synthetic. Natural products are derived from food sources, while synthetic versions are manufactured in laboratories from isolated chemicals. It's a confusing issue, and some consumers believe that they cheat themselves if they "settle" for synthetic vitamins rather than paying more for natural versions.

Despite the hype, natural and synthetic formulations of each nutrient have the same chemical configuration, whether they are obtained from plants or made in a laboratory. Once you remove them from the bottle and swallow them, they act identically in your body. Some "natural" products, in fact, might actually be a combination of a little bit of plant extract and synthetic vitamins; the word *natural* means whatever the manufacturer wants it to mean. But for the most part, both synthetic and natural supplements will provide the nutrients you need—your body won't know the difference.

Be aware that some manufacturers promote their products as originating from various sources—most commonly, vitamin C from "rose hips." In general, you do not need to be concerned about this. As a matter of fact, many "rose hip" vitamins are probably mostly synthetic, with only a small amount of the vitamin C coming from the fleshy base (the "hip") of the rose itself. The rest has been manufactured in a test tube, just like any other synthetic vitamin.

Finally, remember that there is an exception to every rule. Although experts agree that there are no real nutritional differences between synthetic and natural vitamins, it seems that vitamin E may be the exception. Recent research suggests that there *are* clear differences between natural and synthetic vitamin E, and that the natural supplement may be more readily absorbed and used by the body. A study at the National Research Council of Canada, published in the *American Journal of Clinical Nutrition* in 1998, found that "natural vitamin E has roughly twice the availability of synthetic vitamin E." That's a significant difference. But keep in mind that more research needs to be done in this area before firm recommendations can be made about choosing the natural form over the synthetic. Most of the efficacy studies of vitamin E show that the synthetic formulation is effective—although it now seems that the natural E may be even more potent. However, natural vitamin E is more expensive than its synthetic counterpart.

Shopping for Supplements

There's no shortage of places to buy nutritional supplements. They're sold in supermarkets, pharmacies, health food stores, and some department stores. You can even buy your supplements from mail-order houses or on the Internet.

So where should you shop? Except for some variations in price, you may not find much difference among the supplements from one store to another. Only a limited number of companies manufacture vitamins and minerals. These manufacturers supply their brand-name products to outlets throughout the country and also repackage their items with store-brand labels. So while the names on the labels may change, the products are generally identical. Still, just to be safe, it's a good idea to buy supplements at a store known for selling quality merchandise.

A store with a pharmacy inside is one of your best bets when you're choosing supplements. The pharmacist can answer any questions you have about the various products and, if you have any medical problems, can help you choose the product that's best suited to your particular needs.

Understanding Supplement Labels

As with any other product you buy, do some comparison shopping—and not only for price. Read the labels on supplements, and see what you get for your dollar. Look at the description of what's inside the bottle, specifically at the nutrients and their potencies.

Using your personalized program as a guide, you need to determine, for example, if a multivitamin and mineral formulation can give you the amounts of each nutrient that you want. Would you be better off purchasing certain vitamin or mineral supplements individually? The answer may be to combine a broad-spectrum multivitamin and mineral preparation with "booster" doses of selected individual nutrients to meet your particular needs.

Be sure to look carefully at the quantities of nutrients in the bottle. Often you'll find quantities given in milligrams (mg), the equivalent of one-thousandth of a gram. Some vitamins and minerals are needed in such small amounts, however, that they are measured in micrograms (mcg), equal to one-millionth of a gram. Some—such as vitamins A, D, and E—may also be measured in international units (IU), designations of their biological activity, not of their weight. The labels of many products carrying IU values also provide equivalency doses in milligrams or micrograms.

When you consider price, keep in mind not only the number of tablets in the bottle, but also the amount of the nutrient in each tablet. Don't let the size of the bottle or of the capsules themselves deceive you; the quantity of a given vitamin or mineral in a single tablet can differ considerably.

The label may also give you clues about the capacity of the

vitamin or mineral to dissolve in your digestive system and make its way into your bloodstream. The water-soluble vitamins (vitamin C and all of the B vitamins) should dissolve and disintegrate (break into small pieces) in less than an hour. If they don't dissolve this way—and not all pills do—they can't work in your bloodstream. The label probably won't contain this specific information, but look for a designation that the manufacturer adheres to standards created by the U.S. Pharmacopoeia (USP), the scientific body that sets criteria for drug composition. These guidelines require, for example, that water-soluble vitamins disintegrate in the digestive tract within thirty to forty-five minutes. If the label doesn't provide data about the release of the nutrients, or if it doesn't state that the product abides by USP standards, assume that it doesn't meet these guidelines. By the way, no such dissolution test exists yet for the fat-soluble vitamins A, D, E, and K.

Finally, check the expiration date on the label. Don't purchase a product with a date that has already passed or is within a few months of expiring. Look for a product that doesn't expire for several more years.

Using Supplements

Many experts on vitamins and minerals say that your body can make use of supplements no matter what time of day you consume them. If you take them with meals, however, food can often increase the rate at which your intestines absorb them. It might also lessen gastric irritation that may occur if these products are taken on an empty stomach. Also, it's a good idea to take your vitamins and minerals at the same time each day—perhaps with breakfast or dinner—to make it a habit and reduce the chances that you'll forget to take them.

Storing Supplements

Supplements do not remain potent forever. Unopened, vitamins generally last for two or three years. Opened, they may last for about one year. Mineral supplements last longer, and it is not usually the minerals themselves that go bad, but other substances contained in the supplements.

Always store your supplement products away from direct sunlight and heat. A cool, dry place is better than the refrigerator, because the moisture will decrease the potency of certain vitamins and minerals.

SUMMING IT UP

By now you should have a working knowledge of the nature of vitamins and minerals. You understand that these nutrients are essential to life itself because they are involved in *all* of the body's biological processes. And, just as important, you know how to select, use, and store supplement products. But remember that nutritional supplements are just that—supplements. They work best when they are part of a healthful lifestyle.

Armed with this knowledge you are ready to take the first step on the road to optimal health. Read on to learn how herbs can promote health by helping to prevent or fight diseases.

Chapter 2

The Facts About Herbs

For thousands of years, cultures in every area of the world have used herbs for medicinal purposes. In fact, people once consumed entire plants, sensing intuitively that they had health benefits. More recently, scientists have identified the active substances in plants, and have extracted and concentrated them into the herbal products that are now widely available.

In the United States, herbs are gaining newfound respectability, even though they were commonly found on the shelves of most pharmacies until at least fifty years ago. When the first antibiotics were introduced, heralding the beginning of the modern drug age, many herbal remedies were brushed aside by Americans in favor of potent prescription medications. Nevertheless, in a sense, herbs never really left center stage, since about 25 percent of today's conventional drugs actually have their origins in plants. Morphine, for example, is derived from poppies; digitalis, the heart medication, comes from foxglove; and taxol, which is used in cancer therapy, is obtained from the Pacific yew tree. Today, researchers at many pharmaceutical companies are looking to plant life—particularly those plants in the rain forests—as the richest source of future drugs.

Despite their recent resurgence in America, herbs are still more popular in many other countries than they are in the United States. The World Health Organization (WHO) has reported that about 80 percent of the people in the world utilize plants for medicinal purposes, often as their primary form of medication. Even in the more modern areas of Europe, herbal remedies are considered to be either front-line treatments or complements to the best that mainstream medicine can offer. In Germany, for example, about 600 to 700 plant-based remedies are now available, and 70 percent of physicians in that country prescribe them. The use of herbs as remedies has gained greater acceptance in Germany because of the work of a panel called Commission E, a group of physicians, pharmacologists, and scientists appointed by the German Federal Health Agency. The Commission was given the task of creating a collection of reports on the most commonly used herbs, consolidating the credible information about effectiveness, dosing, and possible side effects. At last count, reports on more than 300 herbs had been produced.

Without question, plants can be useful weapons in preventing or fighting diseases. Though herbs are not essential to life, they can promote good health in a number of ways. Consider the following facts:

❑ Studies show that some herbs help strengthen and support the body's immune system. For example, short-term use of echinacea can help the body fight upper respiratory infections.

❑ Research has demonstrated that certain herbs can bolster or complement health-enhancing processes by functioning as antioxidants and supporting the activity of known antioxidant vitamins like C and E. Antioxidants neutralize harmful free radicals that can damage cells in the body.

❑ There is evidence that some herbs can protect human tissue. For instance, saw palmetto can relieve symptoms of prostate enlargement and a condition called benign prostatic hyperplasia.

❑ Investigators have found that some herbs interfere with the development of certain infections. For example, cranberry prevents bacteria from adhering to the wall of the bladder, thereby blocking the bacteria's ability to cause urinary tract infections.

HOW SAFE ARE HERBS?

One appeal of herbs is that they are natural, which most people equate with "safe." Unfortunately, that's not always the case. Herbal remedies have not been subjected to the rigorous testing that drugs must undergo to be approved by the U.S. Food and

Drug Administration. Thus, the safety profiles of herbs—and their effectiveness—have not been as clearly defined as those of FDA-approved drugs.

While most people don't put herbs in the same category as drugs, these plant extracts must not be used indiscriminately. Herbal remedies can be very potent, and some herbs may interact negatively with certain prescription and over-the-counter medications. For example, St. John's wort may interact with some prescription antidepressant medications. So even though herbs are derived from natural plant sources, they must be used with care.

In 1996, the FDA issued warnings about weight-loss products that contained the Chinese herb ma huang, after the agency received reports of negative reactions that included dizziness and seizures. In a few cases, use of the herb even caused death. In 1995, *JAMA (The Journal of the American Medical Association)* reported a case of liver failure in a woman who had used an extract of chaparral, a desert shrub, for ten months. In large amounts, several other herbs—including comfrey root, germander, and Gordoloba yerba tea—have also been associated with liver problems, and herbal preparations containing licorice root have been linked to hypertension (high blood pressure) when taken in large doses.

The most common reactions to herbal preparations include stomach upset, nausea, headaches, and skin rashes. Because herbs are plant material that contains protein, some people also develop allergic symptoms. Nevertheless, for the majority of users, herbs taken in their recommended doses cause few adverse effects, and those that do occur tend to be mild.

Many herbal experts, however, advise pregnant women to use herbs only with the approval of their obstetrician. An herb that is safe for an adult may cause harm to a fetus. Also, as a general rule, breast-feeding mothers, as well as children under the age of six years old, should be given herbal remedies only under the supervision of their doctor. Extensive research has not yet been conducted to evaluate the safety of herbs for these groups.

BUYING HERBS

Herbs are widely available today, not only in health food stores, but also in most pharmacies and supermarkets. They can be purchased as tablets, capsules, teas, tinctures (liquid formulations), and raw seeds and roots.

The quality of herbal preparations is highly variable—that is, the active ingredients of a particular herb may vary from one product to another, or even from one pill to the next in the same product. A recent study of ginseng products, published in the British journal *The Lancet,* reported that some ginseng formulations contain no active ingredients at all!

To be sure you're getting active ingredients in a uniform dose, you need to begin by carefully reading the label of any product that you're considering buying. The label should precisely describe the amount of active ingredients in each dose and provide clear instructions about how much to take.

Look for a product that is *standardized,* which means that each dose contains a precise amount of one or more of the herb's active compounds, usually described as a percentage of the weight of the herbal preparation. For instance, with St. John's wort, the ingredient used as a reference or marker is hypericin, typically in a 0.3-percent concentration. Feverfew is standardized for a constituent called parthenolide, while kava is standardized for active ingredients known as kavalactones. Standardization is a quality control measure designed to ensure batch-to-batch consistency, as well as pharmacological activity. Scan the product label to determine whether a preparation is standardized, and how much of the active constituent is part of each and every dose. Be aware, however, that just because a product is labeled "standardized," there is no guarantee that the label is accurate. Standardization is voluntary for manufacturers, and no external regulating agency monitors the accuracy of such claims. For this and other reasons, I suggest buying herbs from manufacturers with recognizable brand names and well-established reputations. These companies are more likely to take standardization seriously and to have quality control measures in place, which means that they obtain the best available raw materials and test them for the presence of the herb's active constituents, as well as for contaminants. This assures you of consistent quality from box to box or bottle to bottle.

Also, bear in mind that not all herbs are available in standardized form. While herbs such as ginseng, milk thistle, St. John's wort, and ginkgo are widely available in standardized formulations, some other herbs are not sold in standardized preparations. This is because standardization is possible only when an herb's active ingredients are identified and easily measured, which is not the case with certain herbs.

A FINAL WORD

Used appropriately, many herbs can perform healing functions in the body. In fact, some herbal remedies are prescribed almost as often as pharmaceutical products in a number of European countries. More recently, in the United States, a renewed interest in natural healing has sparked scientific research into the health benefits of herbs. As positive evidence about the health-promoting properties of some herbs has accumulated, herbal remedies have become more widely available in pharmacies and health food stores across America.

Nevertheless, remember that the safety and efficacy of many herbal products has not been clearly defined. Herbal remedies can be very potent, and may interact with prescription and over-the-counter medications, so they must be used with care. You'll find guidelines for taking herbal supplements in Chapter 4.

Chapter 3

The Importance of Antioxidants

U ntil recently, much of the medical community had been reluctant to recommend the use of vitamin, mineral, and herbal supplements to promote good health. But a dramatic change in the attitude towards supplementation is occurring, due largely to the impressive evidence about a group of nutrients and herbs known as *antioxidants*. Scientific studies conducted at some of the world's most respected research facilities support the role of these unique nutrients in preventing major chronic diseases and illnesses, from cancer to heart disease to cataracts.

Antioxidants guard the body against highly reactive molecules known as *free radicals*. Uncontrolled, these harmful molecules can wreak havoc on healthy cells and tissues, leading to the development of degenerative diseases. Free-radical damage is also thought to be a major cause of the aging process. By neutralizing free radicals, antioxidants can help put a stop to this cell and tissue damage.

To help you appreciate the role antioxidants play in protecting the body, you'll need to learn a bit about free radicals. This chapter starts with some background on the nature of these potentially harmful molecules.

WHAT ARE FREE RADICALS?

All of your body's cells are made up of atoms that, in turn, contain paired particles called electrons. When every electron in an atom is paired with another electron, the atom is said to be stable. A free radical is an atom or a group of atoms (a molecule) that is short one electron, and is considered to be highly unstable. To regain stability, free radicals attack other molecules in search of an electron— they can target molecules in any cell in the body from which to grab an electron. Every cell in your body is subjected to an esti- mated 10,000 "hits" by free radicals every day. Once a free radical grabs an electron from another molecule, that molecule becomes damaged. Because they join so readily with other molecules, free radicals have the potential to cause a lot of damage.

You may be surprised to learn, then, that the formation of free radicals is a natural consequence of many of the body's biochem- ical processes. For instance, certain immune cells release free radi- cals that can kill invading bacteria and viruses to help prevent infection. Free-radical formation also results from the body's pro- duction of energy. The body uses the macronutrients—carbohy- drates, fats, and proteins—from food in combination with oxygen to produce energy. This process is known as *oxidation.* Although oxidation is fundamental to human survival, an undesirable out- come is the release of oxygen free radicals. To put it simply, we can make this analogy: When your car produces energy from gasoline, a by-product is exhaust, which contains harmful pollutants such as carbon monoxide, sulfur, and nitrogen oxides. In a similar way, when your body uses nutrients and oxygen to produce energy, one outcome is an "exhaust" that contains free radicals.

Under normal circumstances, the body can keep free-radical formation in check, and a reasonable balance can be maintained between the rate of cellular damage and the rate of repair. But sometimes the production of free radicals becomes excessive, upsetting this delicate balance. For example, exposure to chemicals in the air, as well as to radiation from x-rays and cigarette smoke, may cause free-radical formation to become out of control. When the rate of injury to healthy cells and tissues surpasses the rate at which the damage can be repaired, the body is said to be in a state of *oxidative stress.* The body's cells and tissues may not be damaged enough to be considered "sick," but they certainly are not well.

Consider, for example, the oxidative damage and repair that takes place in your body if you exercise too strenuously. The hard- er you exercise, and the more oxygen you take in, the greater the generation of free radicals—and the greater the potential for muscle damage. Free-radical damage is, in part, why you may feel stiff and sore in the days following an intense workout. If you rest for a day or two, your muscles have adequate time to repair themselves, and the pain goes away. Such is the cycle of oxidative stress and cellular healing.

In more extreme cases, however, the damage caused by free radicals may be too extensive to repair. If free radicals attack and damage enough molecules, the onslaught can cause formerly healthy cells to die, and entire organs may be damaged and even cease to work. Free radicals can also alter the body's DNA, which could eventually trigger the development of degenerative diseases such as cancer. Some scientists believe that free radicals contribute significantly to the development of a number of chronic illnesses and to the aging process itself.

Fortunately, our bodies are usually capable of maintaining a healthy balance through cellular repair systems. We also may be able to minimize free-radical damage with antioxidants, which can neutralize free radicals before enough of them accumulate to damage the healthy cells in your body.

WHAT ARE ANTIOXIDANTS?

Antioxidants protect the body against oxidative stress by neutralizing free radicals *before* they can do harm. When an antioxidant encounters a free radical, with its unpaired or missing electron, it gives up one of its own electrons to stabilize the free radical so it is no longer toxic or reactive. As a result, the free radical does not have to seek out and grab an electron from a healthy cell, so it is no longer considered harmful. Also, because antioxidants remain quite stable even after donating their electrons, they become neither toxic nor reactive.

The body manufactures some antioxidants as a matter of course. For example, the enzymes glutathione peroxidase and superoxide dismutase are potent weapons in the body's defense against free radicals. Certain vitamins, minerals, and herbs also have antioxidant effects, particularly vitamins C and E, beta-carotene, zinc, selenium, ginseng, and ginkgo.

Currently, our knowledge is greatest about the antioxidant effects of vitamin C, vitamin E, and beta-carotene. These three micronutrients are found in different parts of the cell; which nutrient is active depends on where a free radical attacks. For example, vitamin E is fat-soluble (dissolves in fat) and is found primarily in cell membranes; it may act most prominently as an antioxidant if damage occurs in the cell membrane. The water-soluble vitamin C is found in the cytoplasm of the cell and may play a more important antioxidant role if a free radical is inside the watery confines of the cell.

ANTIOXIDANTS AND CHRONIC DISEASES

As noted earlier, free radicals have been implicated in the development of some serious degenerative diseases, including cardiovascular disease, which encompasses heart disease and stroke, as well as cancer. Free-radical damage is a contributing factor in the aging process and in the development of conditions associated with aging, such as cataracts. The next few pages explore the ways in which oxidative stress can promote degenerative conditions, so you can better appreciate how antioxidants can help prevent or delay the onset of these and other conditions.

Cardiovascular Disease

The primary cause of cardiovascular disease—including high blood pressure, coronary heart disease (heart attack and angina pectoris, or chest pain), and stroke—is *atherosclerosis*. Atherosclerosis is characterized by the buildup of fat deposits known as plaques along the walls of the arteries. This buildup ultimately causes the passageways of the blood vessels to narrow, making it more difficult for the flow of blood and oxygen to reach the heart muscle and the brain. As more plaque accumulates, the lack of oxygen eventually damages the organs served by the arteries. When blood flow to the heart is cut off, a heart attack occurs; when the brain is affected, a stroke results.

The process that leads to clogged arteries involves numerous factors, some of which are related. Factors that increase the risk of atherosclerosis include: high blood cholesterol, high blood pressure, and smoking. While the blood level of cholesterol plays a major role in the development of atherosclerosis, the action of free radicals on "bad" low-density lipoprotein (LDL) cholesterol also appears to be critical. Research shows that LDL cholesterol is oxidized when attacked by free radicals. Many experts believe that this modification accelerates plaque buildup in the arteries. This may help to explain why cigarette smokers—who have much higher levels of free radicals than nonsmokers—are more likely to suffer heart attacks.

Recent laboratory research has shown that adding the antioxidant vitamin E to plasma decreases the susceptibility of LDL cholesterol to oxidation from free radicals, suggesting that vitamin E may help prevent coronary heart disease in humans. Of thousands of people studied worldwide, those who consumed more antioxidants, either dietary or supplementary, were less likely to develop heart disease. We will look more closely at the results of this research in later chapters on specific antioxidants.

Cancer

The other major life-threatening disease linked to free-radical damage is cancer. While we still do not completely understand the mechanisms involved, many scientists believe that high levels of free radicals may play a role in transforming healthy cells into cancerous cells. Free radicals may be involved in the development of cancers resulting from exposure to cigarette smoke, radiation, and carcinogens (cancer-causing agents) such as asbestos. Some experts think that these cancers result from oxidative damage to DNA, the carrier of genetic material within cells, damaging the DNA in the process. Injury to DNA can result in mutations, which are perpetuated when the DNA replicates within the cells, resulting in mutations that perpetuate the production of abnormal DNA. This may be the first step in what is known to be a long, multistage progression from the initial mutation to a cancerous cell.

Antioxidants seem to help most in preventing cancers linked to free-radical damage—especially those involving the gastrointestinal tract (colon, stomach, esophagus, and oropharynx) and the lungs. Numerous studies have shown that antioxidants can prevent injury to DNA by neutralizing free radicals before they can cause harm. Even after damage has occurred, antioxidants may be able to reverse some of the changes, or at least halt the long progression from simple DNA damage to the development of cancer. However, it is unlikely that the antioxidants can actually reverse the cancer once it has developed.

Eye Disorders

A cataract is an area on the lens of the eye that has become opaque. The lens of the eye is the structure that is responsible for focusing incoming light to form clear images. When proteins in the lens are damaged by chronic exposure to the sun's ultraviolet rays—a potent generator of free radicals—they tend to clump together. This makes the lens opaque, causing blurred vision. The opaque area is a cataract.

Many studies have shown that an increased intake of antioxidants, through dietary or supplementary sources, can reduce the risk of developing cataracts. Since cataract operations are the most common surgical procedure performed in the United States, these research results could have important economic implications, and may also provide tremendous relief from personal stress and inconvenience.

Some eye specialists believe that antioxidants may help prevent an even more serious eye disorder called macular degeneration. This is a condition in which the *macula*—an area of the eye that is responsible for registering fine detail in the center of the field of vision—begins to break down, causing gradual loss of visual acuity. Eventually, the condition can result in severe visual impairment, and it may even lead to permanent blindness.

Macular degeneration is associated with aging, and it affects up to 30 percent of people in the United States aged sixty-five and older. As with cataracts, many experts believe that the disorder may partly result from years of free-radical damage from the sun's ultraviolet rays. If free radicals are involved, antioxidants have the potential to play an important role in protecting the eyes.

Aging and Depressed Immune Function

In the mid-1950s, Dr. Denham Harman suggested that free-radical reactions throughout life could cause the cumulative damage and deficits often associated with aging. Now that we have the technological ability to measure free-radical damage and the effects of antioxidants on free radicals, more physicians are beginning to accept the possibility that Dr. Harman's theory may be correct. Unfortunately, the government's RDAs are not so sensitive to aging concerns. Some guidelines, for instance, give one RDA for people up to the age of fifty and another for those fifty-one and older. Clearly, dividing people into just two groups is a vast over-simplification—a person who is fifty-one years old has very different nutritional needs than someone who is ninety-one years old.

Many laboratory experiments have linked free radicals to the aging-related decline in immune function. Additionally, clinical studies suggest that antioxidants can help slow this rate of immune function decline, and may even reverse it. In fact, studies show that antioxidants may even help reduce the incidence and duration of infection among the elderly by enhancing immunity.

LOOKING TOWARD THE FUTURE

With improving technology and expanding scientific information, researchers are looking to see if free radicals are causing or influencing a wider array of chronic diseases, and if antioxidants could prevent or ameliorate these conditions. Among the diseases being studied are diabetes, Parkinson's disease, and Lou Gehrig's disease. Other studies, such as those on free radicals in relation to exercise-related muscle injuries and the impact of antioxidants on recovery from exercise, may provide insights that will not only help athletes maintain muscle function, but will also keep the aging population active and on the go.

As we improve our understanding of free radicals' role in the development of chronic diseases, and as we increase our knowledge of how antioxidant nutrients can contribute to health, we can provide more specific, targeted recommendations for dietary intakes. You'll learn how to put this information to work in upcoming chapters.

Chapter 4

Developing Your Own Supplement Strategy

Physicians, nutritionists, and researchers agree that a nutrient-poor diet has a negative impact on health, while nutrient-rich foods are important for overall wellness. Unfortunately, good nutrition is often forsaken in the hustle and bustle of our busy world. If you're one of the millions of people who live life in the fast-food lane, you may not be doing everything possible to keep your body functioning at an optimal level.

That's why a vitamin-and-mineral strategy may make sense for you. Of course, even though only 38 percent of the people in the United States say they take vitamins and minerals, in truth, we *all* take these nutrients. Some of us rely exclusively on the foods we eat for our vitamins and minerals; others consider supplements important. Some consume less of the essential nutrients than we need; others take far more than necessary.

The real challenge is to design a supplement program that is unique to your particular needs. How do you know when supplementation is appropriate? Which nutrients do you need to take for optimal health, and in what amounts? Where do herbs fit into your supplement plan?

The answers to these questions are not simple. However, as I spoke to nutrition researchers across the nation while putting together this book, it became clear that no one has to wait years to get the information necessary for making prudent decisions about vitamins and minerals. In fact, enough research has been compiled on many vitamins and minerals for you to make thoughtful, knowledgeable, and safe choices about individual nutrients.

Using the information in this book, you can create your personalized supplement strategy. This chapter will show you how to use the existing research—along with your own good judgment—to determine if you need to take supplements and, if so, which nutrients you should take, and in what quantities.

DETERMINING YOUR NEED FOR SUPPLEMENTS

Vitamin and mineral supplements can provide numerous health benefits for people from all walks of life—and with all sorts of dietary habits—with minimal risk involved. But many people are confused and frustrated by so many contradictory statements about the benefits of nutrient supplementation. Opinions differ as far as specific uses for vitamins and minerals are concerned, and experts disagree about the amounts of these nutrients that should be consumed. Plus, most recommended nutrient intakes don't take into consideration our differences in terms of lifestyle, habits, and overall health. So how do you know whether you're getting enough of the nutrients you need for optimal health?

One of the unique aspects of this book is its personalized nature. As you read through the individual chapters on nutrients, you will learn how to determine your own nutritional needs and how best to meet them. Toward that goal, you need to know the answers to the following questions:

How much of each vitamin and mineral do you need to consume in order to achieve optimal health?

This book includes profiles of each of the major vitamins and minerals. As part of the assessment of each nutrient, you'll find a section titled "Optimal Daily Allowance." This is a careful determination of how much of the nutrient you should take in daily—through diet, supplementation, or a combination of the two—for the healthiest life possible.

For some vitamins and minerals, there is a single recommendation for everyone—a target dose of niacin or vitamin B_6, for example, that will enable you to meet your needs, whether you are in good health or you have minor or even serious health problems. For other nutrients, you'll find a recommended dosage range from which to select the dosage that is most appropriate for your needs, based on your age, sex, and any medical conditions you may have.

The recommended Optimal Daily Allowances of the essential vitamins and minerals are based on the results of scientific studies published in well-respected professional journals. For example, recent studies have clearly proven the value of folic acid in preventing neural tube birth defects. As a result, experts now agree that every woman of childbearing age should take an optimal dose of this B vitamin. Equally persuasive data can help you make decisions about other vitamins and minerals. Recent research has revealed a dramatically reduced risk of heart attack among men and women who supplement their diets with vitamin E. This benefit is achieved primarily by individuals who take in at least 100 international units of vitamin E per day for at least two-and-a-half years. Based on this research, you might be wise to take at least 100 international units per day. This is the kind of information you need to personalize your own supplement strategy.

Do special circumstances in your life affect the amount of a particular vitamin or mineral you need to maintain optimal health?

Certain factors may interfere with your body's ability to absorb and use specific vitamins. For example, some people have trouble digesting milk products, which are a rich source of calcium, vitamin D, and other nutrients. Individuals who suffer from intestinal disorders may need to consume more of the fat-soluble vitamins A, D, E, and K because their bodies can't absorb these nutrients efficiently. And people who smoke cigarettes require at least twice as much vitamin C as nonsmokers. This is just a small sample of the factors that affect nutrient absorption and use by the body. When you are provided with a recommended dosage range for a given vitamin, use the risk-related information to select your personal optimal intake.

In cases where a single dose is recommended, that level should be high enough to compensate for increased risks based on lifestyle or on any illnesses you may have. The single recommended dose will not only prevent deficiencies and make up for special medical conditions, but it will also help you attain an optimal level of health.

Can you take in the Optimal Daily Allowance of a given vitamin or mineral through diet alone?

It is possible to obtain your entire recommended intake of certain vitamins and minerals from dietary sources. For instance, the Optimal Daily Allowance (ODA) of vitamin A is 1,000 micrograms of RE (retinol equivalents), or 5,000 international units. A one-cup serving of cantaloupe pieces contains 516 micrograms of vitamin A, providing about half of your total needs for the day. A single medium-sized carrot—containing 2,025 micrograms—or one sweet potato—with 2,488 micrograms—easily provides more than the optimal amount. In addition to the ODA of vitamin A, you'll find a separate ODA of mixed carotenoids, which are important antioxidants and precursors of vitamin A. Again, a carrot or two can meet the needs of most people. Clearly, you can achieve the Optimal Daily Allowance of some important micronutrients simply by making wise food choices.

However, this is not so easy for a nutrient such as vitamin E. Ideally, you should take several times more of this important vitamin than the government's guidelines suggest. Although the RDA of vitamin E is 15 international units per day for men, and even less for nonpregnant women, I recommend that *all* adults get at least 100 international units per day. To take in the RDA for men, you'd have to eat 32 medium-sized apricots, 48 dried prunes, 3 cups of walnuts, or 3.3 tablespoons of oil-and-vinegar dressing per day! To meet the ODA, you'd need to consume even larger quantities of food—212 apricots, 317 prunes, 18 cups of walnuts, 22 tablespoons of oil-and-vinegar dressing, or a combination of these or similar foods. Obviously, that's just not practical.

HOW TO DESIGN YOUR NUTRITIONAL SUPPLEMENT PROGRAM

There are a lot of factors to consider when you develop your individualized supplement program. Your nutritional needs are unique to you, so a program that works for someone else might not meet your needs. To design a nutritional supplement program that is suited to your particular requirements, keep the following strategies in mind as you read through the individual chapters on vitamins and minerals.

STRATEGY 1

The goal of vitamin and mineral intake is not just to prevent deficiency diseases, but to achieve a state of optimal health. Aim to take in enough of the nutrients you need for maximum well-being, rather than taking supplements to avoid deficiencies.

For decades, most recommendations for vitamin and mineral intake have been based on the lowest level necessary to prevent deficiency symptoms, with a modest margin of safety added. The scientific panel that sets RDAs recently stated that its recommendations are for "the levels of intake of essential nutrients that, on the basis of scientific knowledge, are judged by the Food and Nutrition Board to be adequate to meet the known nutrient needs of practically all healthy persons." The panel stated that it was impossible to determine and establish "optimal" doses higher than the RDAs.

This approach is far from ideal, however. First, many people are not "healthy"—a term that's defined differently by just about everyone, anyway. The RDAs may be much too low for people who have medical disorders, such as diabetes or kidney disease, for those who use alcohol or certain medications, and for persons who have unusual dietary patterns. Some of these individuals should take many times the RDA of specific nutrients to compensate for their particular circumstances.

Also, despite what RDA panelists have said, strong evidence now suggests that larger doses of certain nutrients can do far more than simply prevent deficiency diseases. Increased amounts of selected vitamins and minerals may help prevent some of the conditions of aging that were once considered inevitable, which will be discussed in greater detail in later chapters. To the extent you can potentially benefit from larger doses, it makes sense to increase doses—provided the monetary cost is reasonable and the potential risk of adverse reactions is low. Most people should probably take more than the RDAs of many vitamins and minerals.

Fortunately, the federal government is committed to updating the RDAs, one by one, although the process is moving forth slowly. They have already done so with several nutrients. For example:

❏ The RDA of folic acid was recently increased from 180 to 400 micrograms. Yet, right up until the time the RDA was raised, most experts insisted that 180 micrograms was enough. Now we know it was too low—and that some babies may have been born with spina bifida because it took so long to recognize what the research was showing.

❏ The RDA of vitamin D (200 to 400 international units for most adults) was recently raised for several population groups, including the elderly and those who are confined indoors. Now, the panel tells us that these new levels are essential; not long ago, they were equally insistent that the lower amounts were just fine.

❏ The calcium guidelines have been raised to as high as 1,500 milligrams for some women to avoid osteoporosis. The same panel that just raised the recommended intake told us in the mid-1990s that 1,000 milligrams was enough.

STRATEGY 2

For each nutrient, the optimal dose should balance the maximum benefits with the minimum potential risk. As with most things in life, the goal of nutritional planning is to gain the greatest possible good without putting yourself in jeopardy. So whenever potential benefits of higher vitamin or mineral levels outweigh potential risks, increasing your intake makes sense.

Unfortunately, the situation is not always clear-cut. At low doses, the benefits generally do outweigh the risks. But the medical literature is filled with reports of dangerous side effects for some nutrients when they are taken at extremely high doses. Unfortunately, few statistically sound studies have accurately weighed the risks and benefits of higher intake levels of most vitamins and minerals.

Because of the fear of adverse effects, many physicians and nutritional experts continue to recommend the relatively conservative RDAs for all vitamins and minerals. But this matter can be approached differently. It is true that levels at or near the RDAs make sense for selected nutrients whose toxic levels can be reached fairly quickly, particularly when no clear evidence indicates that larger doses offer additional health benefits. But the reverse also holds true. For vitamin E, for example, research strongly suggests major benefits from larger doses, and no significant side effects have been found among people who have taken these increased doses for long periods of time. Therefore, it makes sense to boost your intake of vitamin E to the ODA level.

If a situation is unclear, the prudent course is to take the lower doses until evidence indicates either that higher levels are risk-free or that higher levels confer sufficient additional benefits to warrant some risks. The information in this book will help you make these decisions.

STRATEGY 3

When appropriate, personalize your strategy to meet your unique needs in terms of age, sex, size, lifestyle, and medical condition. The individual vitamin and mineral chapters in this book will guide you in deciding if you need extra amounts of particular nutrients because of your unique circumstances. For other vitamins and minerals, a single recommended dose is appropriate for everyone, making up for deficiencies and shortcomings and promoting optimal health.

STRATEGY 4

Use foods as your source of vitamins and minerals whenever possible. A varied and balanced diet will provide your body with a variety of the vitamins and minerals you need, without any risk of side effects. And keep in mind that foods supply you with other important substances that you can't get from a supplement—from energy-producing proteins and carbohydrates to cholesterol-lowering fibers.

However, you may not be able to get enough of the necessary nutrients through foods alone. If you're on a low-calorie diet for weight loss, if your body does not tolerate dairy products, or if a chronic disease interferes with your body's absorption of nutrients, for example, you will need to supplement your meals with vitamin and mineral pills.

STRATEGY 5

Use vitamins and minerals to complement a healthful lifestyle—not to compensate for unhealthful habits. Some people believe they can make up for all kinds of undesirable behaviors by taking vitamin and mineral supplements. But a supplement certainly can't replace the cardiovascular and many other benefits of exercise. And while vitamins, minerals, or herbs may help overcome free-radical formation stimulated by cigarette smoking, they won't protect you from nicotine's destructive effects upon your heart. In the same way, if you eat a lot of high-fat foods or have other unhealthful habits, a few vitamin and mineral capsules won't rescue you from a health crisis at some point in your life. Nutritional supplements should be an adjunct to the other health-enhancing behaviors that are part of your day-to-day living.

WHAT ABOUT HERBS?

In Part Four, you will find individual chapters on seventeen of the most popular herbs available today. Although the information on the potential health benefits of herbs is less extensive than that for vitamins and minerals, ongoing studies of many of these medicinal plants have thus far yielded promising results. While these botanicals are not essential to life itself, scientific research has revealed what many traditional cultures have believed for centuries—that many plants have medicinal properties. Herbs contain active constituents that may strengthen the body's defenses or maintain the health of the body and mind.

If you decide to try any of the herbs described in this book, keep the following points in mind. First, even though herbs are "natural" and often have beneficial properties, they nevertheless may have side effects. Therefore, herbal remedies must be used appropriately, not indiscriminately. Some herbs should not be used for extended periods of time. Others are safe enough to become an integral part of your regular supplement program. Make sure that you are aware of the benefits and risks of taking any herbal product, and take only the recommended dosage for the suggested length of time. Also, since herbs contain active ingredients, they should be used with caution in conjunction with prescribed drugs.

If you regularly take any kind of medication, check with your doctor before undertaking an herbal treatment program, as some herbs may interact negatively with pharmaceutical products.

Finally, use common sense when it comes to taking any herbal preparation. Pay close attention to how it makes you feel. Although most people do not experience side effects, some may show sensitivity to particular herbs, and could experience symptoms such as headaches, stomach upset, and nausea.

WORKING WITH YOUR HEALTH-CARE PRACTITIONER

Most physicians make few, if any, recommendations to their patients about using supplements of vitamins, minerals, and herbs, and some—surprisingly—still discourage their use altogether. A 1998 Gallup survey revealed that only 19 percent of American physicians even discussed supplementation with their patients, and a significant proportion of those who did actually advised their patients not to take any supplements. That kind of recommendation is startling, considering the available evidence supporting the use of some nutrient supplements, such as folic acid for *all* women of childbearing age.

When you talk with your own physician, here are some ideas to keep in mind:

❑ Always let the doctor know what you are already taking. As "good-for-you" as nutritional supplements may seem, some can interact adversely with certain drugs and can cause potentially dangerous side effects. Some people may also experience allergic reactions to some supplements.

❑ If your physician has an across-the-board policy of "Don't take supplements," regardless of your dietary habits, you need to look for a doctor who understands the need to personalize nutrition advice. Along these lines, if your physician advises against supplements, but you fall into a population group where supplementation makes sense—(e.g., you are a woman of childbearing age)—find another doctor who is familiar with the current science in the nutritional field.

❑ Make sure your doctor customizes his or her supplement recommendations to fit your age, sex, and medical needs. For example, menstruating women need more iron than women after menopause; men tend to require more B vitamins than women because of their greater muscle mass and carbohydrate intake; people at high risk for heart disease may need more vitamin E and other antioxidants than those at low risk; and so forth.

If you are interested in taking herbal supplements to improve your overall health or to treat a specific condition, you may be reluctant to discuss your decision with your health-care practitioner. Perhaps you think that your doctor is unfamiliar with herbs, or that he or she will disapprove of using herbs because they are not FDA-approved. But despite these hesitations, it's extremely important that you let your doctor know about the herbs you're taking, and even those herbs you're thinking about using. Before attempting to self-treat an illness or condition—particularly a serious one—it is crucial to have the proper diagnosis. A physician who is familiar with herbs will also know whether a particular physical condition precludes the use of certain herbal preparations.

Once you begin using an herb, be aware of the possibility of negative reactions. If you experience any side effects when you start taking a new herb, you should stop using it and see if the symptoms subside. If the reaction is severe, contact your physician immediately.

HOW TO USE THIS BOOK

Now that we've covered the basics, we're ready to move on to the individual chapters on vitamins, minerals, and herbs. In Parts Two and Three, you will learn the important information you need to know about vitamins and minerals, including how these nutrients function in the body, who's at risk of deficiency, and how to recognize symptoms of deficiency and toxicity. Remember, for each individual nutrient, you will find an Optimal Daily Allowance—in some cases a suggested ODA range—along with an explanation of why this dosage has been recommended.

The individual chapters on herbs will tell you what you should know about using herbs to enhance your health. Each chapter provides interesting background and historical information on herbal remedies, including their traditional use throughout the ages. Then you'll learn a bit about the most important active constituents contained in the herbs, and how they work to strengthen and heal the body. The individual chapters will also provide you with a recommended dosage that is safe and effective for most people, and crucial information about safety and adverse effects.

On the illness-to-wellness continuum, you should strive to move as far to the wellness end of the spectrum as possible. The information in this book will guide you in creating a sound supplement strategy that can help you achieve that goal.

Part Two

The Vitamins

Chapter 5

Vitamin A

Vitamin A has numerous and diverse functions in the body, but it may be best known for the role it plays in preventing night blindness and other eye problems. It also helps to promote and maintain healthy immune system function; it is essential for cellular growth and development; and it is needed for healthy skin and hair. And, as you learned in Chapter 3, vitamin A functions as an antioxidant, so it helps protect body cells and tissues against cardiovascular disease and cancer, which are believed to be linked to free-radical damage.

Vitamin A is actually a group of compounds that are structurally related and have a similar biological activity. These compounds can be divided into two categories: the *retinoids* (preformed vitamin A) and the *carotenoids* (precursors of vitamin A). The retinoids are considered "active" forms of vitamin A because the body can use them immediately upon consumption. *Retinol* is the principal retinoid.

The carotenoids are the yellow-red plant pigments commonly found in fruits and vegetables such as sweet potatoes, apricots, cantaloupes, and carrots. They got their name in the 1930s, when they were first discovered in carrots. Today, more than 500 of these compounds have been identified. Some carotenoids are converted to active vitamin A in the body, and some act as antioxidants. *Beta-carotene* is the best known of the carotenoids.

The retinoids occur naturally in animal sources, while the carotenoids are produced only by plants. To meet your body's vitamin A requirements, you can consume either preformed retinoids or carotenoids such as beta-carotene. Like vitamin A itself, beta-carotene is fat-soluble. The carotenoids have a distinct advantage because they do not appear to cause toxicity, which is a known danger of consuming too much preformed vitamin A. Plus, the body can decrease its conversion of beta-carotene to vitamin A when blood levels of vitamin A are high, so even when you increase your intake of beta-carotene, your body's conversion process automatically slows down.

FUNCTIONS IN THE BODY

Vitamin A is essential for healthy eyes. It helps form the pigments in the eye that allow proper functioning of the light-sensitive *retina*—hence, the name *retinoids*. Each time the eyes are exposed to light, a little of the vitamin A-rich compounds in these pigments is used, and more of the nutrient is needed to regenerate the supply. Without enough vitamin A, vision in dim light worsens and you experience night blindness.

The History of Vitamin A

Scientists have known of the existence of vitamin A for centuries, although the nutrient acquired its name relatively recently. More than 3,500 years ago, some civilizations had already discovered a connection between night blindness and a deficiency in foods that we now know are rich in vitamin A. Egyptian documents traced back to 1500 BC describe treating night blindness by squeezing the juice from roasted or fried animal liver directly onto the eyes. During the third and fourth centuries BC, Hippocrates suggested including liver in the diet to treat night blindness. Today, we know that liver is particularly rich in vitamin A.

Early in the twentieth century, researchers working with animals determined that specific nutritional substances were necessary for growth and survival. These studies showed that at least one of the substances—later identified as vitamin A—could be found in foods such as egg yolks and cod liver oil. A Swiss scientist first described the precise structure of vitamin A in 1930.

Another vital function of vitamin A is its role in the normal growth and maintenance of the epithelial tissues, which include the skin and all of the protective linings of the trachea, the lungs, and the digestive, reproductive, and urinary tracts. In the case of vitamin A deficiency, these tissues will stop producing mucus (the substance that helps preserve and lubricate the body) and instead begin secreting a hard protein called *keratin*. This dries out and toughens the epithelial tissues and makes the body more vulnerable to infections.

Vitamin A can make the immune system more responsive, thus improving the body's resistance to infection and perhaps to diseases such as cancer. Research has shown that vitamin A therapy can reduce deaths from measles and respiratory illnesses, for example. This protective effect is probably at least partly based on vitamin A's role in maintaining the health of the skin and other natural barriers that can keep out infection.

A number of studies have shown that a high intake of vitamin A and/or the carotenoids may help reduce the risk of cancer. This benefit seems to be related to several properties that vitamin A and the carotenoids possess. As discussed above, vitamin A helps strengthen the immune system, and also keeps epithelial tissues healthy, thus interfering with the process by which many cancers develop. Plus, the carotenoids function as antioxidants, which can neutralize the free radicals that have been implicated in the development of some cancers. However, more studies are needed to prove conclusively that vitamin A and the carotenoids can provide this protective effect.

In both men and women, vitamin A promotes the normal workings of the reproductive system. It is also important for a healthy pregnancy and for lactation, although the reasons for this are still unclear.

The presence of vitamin A also appears to be necessary for the normal growth and development of bones, although its role in this process is not well understood.

HEALTH BENEFITS

The body of evidence supporting the health benefits of vitamin A and beta-carotene—a precursor of vitamin A—is growing rapidly.

Many benefits are related to the role of vitamin A, regardless of its source, in the body's biochemical and physiological processes at a cellular level. Others have to do with the antioxidant powers of beta-carotene.

Cancer

The results of numerous studies have indicated that beta-carotene may provide protection against cancer, particularly cancers of the lungs, stomach, breast, cervix, and mouth. However, some recent research has raised doubts about the nutrient's effectiveness as a preventive agent against certain types of cancer, especially lung cancer.

Lung Cancer

One of the earliest and most persuasive studies concerning the effectiveness of carotenes in preventing lung cancer was a nineteen-year evaluation of 1,954 middle-aged employees of the Western Electric Company in Chicago. Researchers found that individuals who consumed the least amount of carotenes were seven times more likely to develop lung cancer than individuals who consumed the greatest amount of carotenes. Of the thirty-three men who developed lung cancer during this study, twenty-five were in the lower half of the range for carotene intake. It's important to note that preformed vitamin A did not decrease the risk of developing lung cancer—the benefits were derived solely from carotene intake.

A study published in 1991 by researchers at Johns Hopkins University also highlighted the possibilities that beta-carotene offers for lung cancer prevention. Starting in 1974, the researchers collected and froze blood samples of some 25,000 residents of Washington County, Maryland. During the next fifteen years, the researchers measured the levels of antioxidants in the blood samples, and compared these levels in the ninety-nine people who had developed lung cancer with those of individuals who remained cancer-free. On average, the blood levels of beta-carotene in individuals with cancer were 16 percent lower than they were in the participants who did not develop cancer. The researchers concluded that the individuals who had the lowest blood levels of beta-carotene were 2.2 times more likely to develop lung cancer than those with the highest levels of the antioxidant.

Two other studies concerning vitamin A and lung cancer are also important. In 1994, researchers at the U.S. National Cancer Institute and the National Public Health Institute in Finland reported their conclusions on an extended study of 29,133 Finnish men. In the study, the participants—all long-term smokers—were divided into four groups: The members of the first group took 20 milligrams of beta-carotene each day; those in the second group supplemented with 50 milligrams of vitamin E each day; individuals in the third group took both vitamins in the same amounts; and members of the fourth group took a placebo, with no active ingredients. Surprisingly, the researchers found that beta-carotene and vitamin E do not offer smokers any protection against lung cancer. Even more startling was the suggestion that beta-carotene *increased* the risk of lung cancer among cigarette smokers by 18 percent. Other findings of the study suggested a rise in the risk of heart disease and stroke in the group that supplemented with beta-carotene, alone or with vitamin E. The authors of the study could not explain these troubling results, particularly those surrounding the increased risk of lung cancer associated with the use of beta-carotene, which had always been considered a safe supplement. An editorial accompanying the study pointed out that the conclusions about lung cancer ". . . may simply have been due to an extreme play of chance, since the finding is so much at variance with the totality of other evidence suggesting a benefit." This is certainly a possibility.

Two years later, in 1996, researchers at the Fred Hutchinson Cancer Research Center in Seattle reported some additional surprising results. This placebo-controlled study, which involved more than 18,000 participants—all current or former smokers or workers exposed to asbestos—analyzed the effects of daily supplementation with 25,000 international units of vitamin A plus 30 milligrams of beta-carotene on the incidence of lung cancer. After four years of follow-up, the study was terminated prematurely because of its unsettling findings. Results showed that individuals supplementing with vitamin A and beta-carotene had a 28 percent greater risk of developing lung cancer than individuals taking a placebo. The group taking the vitamins also had a 26 percent higher likelihood of dying from cardiovascular disease. Keep in mind, however, that the participants in this study already had an elevated risk of lung cancer and cardiovascular problems because of smoking or exposure to asbestos.

While the results of two studies—no matter how large or carefully conducted—should not undermine all of the favorable evidence from the research that has preceded them, this recent research cannot be overlooked. Many of the early studies on beta-carotene were highly persuasive; of some 200 published reports, the majority have shown that the nutrient offers positive benefits. However, these two recent studies highlight the need for continued research on beta-carotene and its effects on lung cancer before any definite conclusions can be reached.

Other Forms of Cancer

Research on the effects of beta-carotene on other forms of cancer has also produced mostly positive results. For example, one study conducted in Switzerland tracked 2,974 men over a period of twelve years. The results, published in 1991, showed that men with low blood levels of carotenoids had a higher death rate from cancer. This seemed to be particularly true of stomach cancer—carotene levels were nearly 60 percent higher in survivors than they were in participants who died of stomach cancer.

A study conducted by researchers at the Fred Hutchinson Cancer Research Center and the University of Washington, Seattle showed a positive correlation between high beta-carotene intake and a reduced incidence of cervical cancer. In this study, the diets of 189 women diagnosed with cancer of the cervix were analyzed and compared with the diets of a control group of 227 cancer-free women. The researchers reported in 1989 that high intakes of beta-carotene were associated with a reduced risk of developing cervical cancer. On the other hand, the intake of preformed vitamin A showed no protective effect against this form of cancer.

In a study conducted in Britain, blood samples from 5,004 women were drawn and frozen, and the health of the women was monitored for several years. During the course of the study, thirty-nine of the participants developed breast cancer. Then, in 1984, researchers from St. Bartholomew's Hospital in London evaluated the original blood samples. The researchers reported that blood levels of beta-carotene in the women without cancer were nearly 50 percent higher than the levels in women with breast cancer.

Researchers at the University of Arizona examined the effects of high doses of beta-carotene on precancerous lesions of the mouth known as *leukoplakia*. They treated twenty-four patients with 30 milligrams of beta-carotene daily for three to six months each. The results of their study, published in 1991, reported that leukoplakia lesions regressed partially or completely in 71 percent of these patients.

While these reports all seem very promising, it must be noted that some studies of beta-carotene's effects on other types of cancer did not produce positive results. For instance, in 1996, researchers at Harvard University published a large-scale study tracking the health of 22,000 male physicians, forty to eighty-four years old, who supplemented with beta-carotene. For this study, half of the participants took 50 milligrams of supplemental beta-carotene every other day, while the other half took a placebo. Twelve years later, the cancer rates were virtually identical in the two groups, showing that supplementation with beta-carotene did not have a significant effect on the incidence of any particular cancer, including lung cancer. In this same study, the researchers also evaluated the effect of supplementation with beta-carotene on cardiovascular disease. The results of their research are discussed below.

Cardiovascular Disease

The findings of several major studies suggest that beta-carotene may help decrease the risk of cardiovascular disease. However, as with the studies of beta-carotene's effects on cancer, some recent research has raised doubts about the antioxidant's protective benefits. Experts must await the results of ongoing studies before drawing any conclusions.

Since 1980, researchers at Harvard University have been monitoring the health of 87,245 female nurses. In 1991, the researchers reported that high beta-carotene intake is associated with a decreased risk of heart attack. The women who consumed the most beta-carotene had 22 percent fewer heart attacks than the participants who consumed the least amounts.

In another Harvard study, beginning in 1982, researchers have been tracking the health of nearly 40,000 male physicians, forty to seventy-five years old. At the start of the study, 333 participants had already been identified as having heart disease, and had previously undergone angioplasty or coronary bypass surgery. According to data published in 1990, among the 333 men, those taking a 50-milligram supplement of beta-carotene every other day had a 44 percent lower risk of having a major cardiovascular event, such as a heart attack or stroke, compared with the men who took a placebo.

Researchers conducting a study in the Boston area closely monitored the heart health of nearly 1,300 older men and women for close to five years. The results of their research, published in 1992, showed that the individuals who consumed the greatest amounts of beta-carotene had a 75 percent lower risk of suffering a fatal heart attack than the participants who consumed the smallest amounts.

In 1994, *JAMA (The Journal of the American Medical Association)* published the findings of a study involving approximately 3,800 men with high cholesterol. Researchers measured levels of carotenoids in blood samples from the participants, and evaluated the correlation between carotenoid levels in the blood and the risk of coronary heart disease (CHD). They reported that men with the highest levels of carotenoids were 36 percent less likely to develop CHD than men with the lowest levels.

Researchers at the National Institute of Public Health in the Netherlands found that people who consumed higher levels of beta-carotene were less likely to suffer a stroke. Beginning in 1960, the investigators took careful dietary histories of a group of 552 men to determine how much beta-carotene they regularly consumed. Over the course of the next fifteen years, the researchers closely monitored the health of the participants. They found that men with the highest intakes of beta-carotene were 46 percent less likely to have a stroke during the fifteen-year follow-up period than their counterparts who consumed the least amounts of carotenoids.

In contrast to the encouraging studies like these, other published research has found that beta-carotene offers no protection against cardiovascular disease. A study conducted in Finland, published in 1996, examined the effects of certain antioxidants on more than 22,000 male smokers, none of whom showed evidence of coronary disease. The volunteers were divided into four groups: Men in the first group supplemented with 20 milligrams per day of beta-carotene; those in the second group took 50 milligrams per day of vitamin E; individuals in the third group supplemented with both beta-carotene and vitamin E; and those in the fourth group took a placebo, with no active ingredients. After about five years, close to 2,000 of the volunteers had developed angina, or chest pain. No evidence indicated, however, that beta-carotene decreased the likelihood of angina; in fact, the incidence actually increased slightly in the men supplementing with beta-carotene alone. Interestingly, vitamin E reduced the incidence of angina by 9 percent.

Another blow to the case for beta-carotene was the Harvard University study first discussed on page 53. As you'll recall, this study involved more than 22,000 male physicians. Half of the group took 50 milligrams of supplemental beta-carotene every other day, while the other half took a placebo. After twelve years, there were virtually no differences between the two groups—that is, the beta-carotene supplements did not provide protection against heart attacks, or death from heart disease or stroke. However, supplementation with the antioxidant did not appear to *increase* the risk of cardiovascular disease, either. Of the participants, 468 men taking beta-carotene suffered heart attacks over the study period, compared with 489 in the placebo group—a difference that was not statistically significant. Rates of death from cardiovascular disease were also statistically similar—338 in the beta-carotene group compared with 313 in the placebo group.

HIV Infection

Vitamin A and beta-carotene may offer some hope for individuals whose immune system function is impaired, particularly people with acquired immune deficiency syndrome, more commonly known as AIDS.

Researchers at Johns Hopkins University compared vitamin A levels in 126 individuals who tested positive for human immunodeficiency virus (HIV), which causes AIDS, and 53 who tested negative but who were considered at high risk of HIV infection. The results of the study, published in 1993, revealed that those people who tested negative for infection with the virus had blood levels of vitamin A that were about 25 percent higher than levels in the people who tested positive. Among the HIV-positive group, deaths in subsequent years were six times greater in vitamin A-deficient individuals than in individuals with adequate intakes of the vitamin. The researchers concluded that vitamin A is a necessary nutrient for normal functioning of the immune system, and that a deficiency of this vitamin "seems to be an important risk factor for disease progression" in HIV infection.

Eye Disorders

Researchers have found that beta-carotene has a protective effect against common eye disorders such as cataracts and macular degeneration. A study conducted in 1991 at Tufts University and other Boston-area institutions looked at blood levels of carotenes in seventy-seven men and women with cataracts, and thirty-five men and women who did not have cataracts. The study revealed that the risk of developing cataracts was significantly higher in individuals with low blood levels of beta-carotene. Participants in the lowest 20 percent for blood beta-carotene levels were five times more likely to develop cataracts than individuals in the top 20 percent.

Researchers in Finland examined forty-seven men and women with cataracts and ninety-four cataract-free men and women. The participants ranged in age from forty to eighty-three years old. According to data published in 1992, researchers at the University of Tampere found that both men and women whose blood levels of beta-carotene measured in the lowest third of the group had a 70 percent higher risk of developing cataracts, compared with people in the remaining two-thirds of the group.

As we first discussed on page 30, the aging-related condition known as macular degeneration is the gradual breakdown of the macula in the eye (the part of the retina responsible for producing detailed images), which can result in severe visual impairment. It is the leading cause of blindness in people sixty-five years of age and older. Researchers have examined the theory that oxidative damage to the macula causes or contributes to this breakdown. In

1993, researchers conducted a study, involving more than 1,000 individuals, to examine the antioxidant benefits of beta-carotene in preventing macular degeneration. The results, published in the *Archives of Ophthalmology,* showed that individuals with the highest blood levels of carotenoids were only one-third as likely to develop macular degeneration as those with the lowest carotenoid levels.

DEFICIENCY SYMPTOMS

Vitamin A can be stored in the liver and released into the bloodstream for use by the body as needed, so we don't need to consume vitamin A every day to prevent signs of deficiency. For that reason, *occasional* dietary deficiencies will probably not cause major deficiency symptoms. However, chronic vitamin A deficiency can cause obvious deficiency symptoms, some of them serious.

Night blindness is an early and reversible symptom of vitamin A deficiency (see page 48). But a severe or long-term deficiency can also potentially cause irreversible damage to the eyes. Chronic deficiency can lead to a drying of the eyes, called *xerosis,* which may cause ulcerations of the cornea.

Because of vitamin A's role in strengthening immunity, a deficiency of this nutrient can increase the body's vulnerability to certain types of infections, particularly in the respiratory tract. Sore throats, sinus infections, and ear infections may occur more frequently if inadequate levels of vitamin A are present.

Vitamin A deficiency can also interfere with normal growth in children. Because the vitamin helps bones develop normally, when it is deficient, bone growth is impaired. Rapid weight loss can occur as well.

In a condition known as *follicular hyperkeratosis,* the body's epithelial tissues produce too much keratin. When this happens in the skin, goosebump-like deposits of keratin form around the hair follicles, typically on the shoulders, neck, back, buttocks, arms, and legs. Eventually, as the condition worsens, the skin assumes a rough texture. Excessive keratin production may also involve the epithelial cells of vital internal organs. In the respiratory tract, mucous secretions essential for carrying foreign bodies out of the lungs may decline. If the nose and mouth are affected, the senses of smell and taste can be lost. Loss of appetite and weight loss also appear to be related to keratinization of the tongue.

Deficiency-related problems of reproduction may involve decreased ability of the body to manufacture sperm, spontaneous abortion (miscarriage), abnormal menstruation, or birth defects.

TOXICITY SYMPTOMS

When vitamin A is consumed in excess of the body's needs, the extra is stored in the liver, providing a ready reserve for days when too little vitamin A is taken in. About 90 percent of the vitamin A present in the body is stored in the liver. When the liver reaches its storage capacity, however, blood levels of the vitamin begin to rise. Excessive amounts of vitamin A, taken over an extended period of time, can accumulate in the liver and in the blood, and can eventually reach toxic levels.

When toxicity does occur, it is usually the result of too many vitamin A supplements. Few foods contain enough preformed vitamin A to cause toxicity symptoms when consumed in normal amounts. One of the best-known exceptions is liver—but few people eat enough liver for problems to occur.

In the early stages, signs of vitamin A toxicity include blurred vision, drowsiness, headache, irritability, loss of appetite, muscular weakness, and scaling or peeling of the skin. Chronic high levels of vitamin A can cause bone pain, diarrhea, edema, fissures of the lips, hair loss, itching, lethargy, menstrual irregularity, weight loss, and enlargement of the liver and the spleen.

Elderly people seem to have an increased risk of developing toxicity symptoms, compared with young or middle-aged adults. This most likely results from decreased clearance of vitamin A from the blood that is associated with advancing age.

Infants and children tend to be far more susceptible than adults to problems associated with excessive vitamin A intake; youngsters typically experience toxic symptoms at much lower doses, and their symptoms are likely to be more pronounced. Some of the early symptoms of vitamin A toxicity in children—including irritability and loss of appetite—are similar to those in adults. Infants and children may also feel lethargic. In infants, an additional sign

Are You at Risk of Vitamin A Deficiency?

How do you know if you're at risk of vitamin A deficiency? Take a moment to review the questions below. If you answer yes to any of these questions, you have an above-average risk of developing a deficiency.

❏ *Do you have chronic liver disease?* The efficient storage of vitamin A in the body relies on the health of the liver. Therefore, liver diseases—including hepatitis, cirrhosis, and liver cancer—can reduce the amount of vitamin A stored by the body.

❏ *Do you have chronic diarrhea?* This condition reduces the absorption of vitamin A, so your body can't effectively use the vitamin A that you take in through dietary sources or supplementation.

❏ *Do you take cholesterol-lowering medications?* Cholesterol-lowering agents—including cholestyramine and colestipol—can diminish the body's ability to absorb vitamin A in the intestinal tract.

❏ *Do you use mineral oil as a laxative?* The use of mineral oil may cause vitamin A deficiency because fat-soluble vitamins are dissolved in the indigestible oil and are excreted.

❏ *Do you take oral contraceptives?* Oral contraceptives cause extra vitamin A to be released from the liver into the bloodstream, which may increase the body's need for vitamin A by decreasing stores in the liver.

❏ *Do you drink large amounts of alcohol?* Alcohol reduces levels of vitamin A in the liver. Also, alcoholics tend to substitute alcohol—which has no real nutritional value—for nutrient-dense foods, so they generally don't take in adequate amounts of vitamin A and other nutrients.

❏ *Do you smoke cigarettes?* Cigarette smoking decreases the level of beta-carotene in the blood.

❏ *Are you under a great deal of physical or emotional stress?* Stress can reduce blood levels of the retinol form of vitamin A, most likely by increasing the body's production of free radicals. Stress may also increase the rate of vitamin A breakdown in the body.

❏ *Are you pregnant or breast-feeding?* Pregnancy is a time of increased nutritional needs because the growth of a new person requires every known nutrient. Women who are breast-feeding should also take in adequate vitamin A to compensate for the amount that is contained in breast milk.

is bulging of the fontanel—the soft spot on the top of an infant's skull. Long-term toxic levels of vitamin A can result in bone pain, premature bone closure, and stunted growth.

Pregnant women should take vitamin A only under the supervision of a doctor, since large doses have been associated with spontaneous abortion (miscarriage) and birth defects, including malformation of the head, face, heart, or nervous system. The risks of vitamin A toxicity to pregnant women were demonstrated in a study conducted at Boston University in 1995. In that study of almost 23,000 pregnancies, investigators found that the chances of birth defects increased when women took more than 10,000 international units of vitamin A per day early in their pregnancy. The study concluded that one in fifty-seven babies born to women taking these high doses—more than twice the RDA for pregnant women—would have one of the birth defects listed above. However, the researchers noted that beta-carotene seemed to be quite safe and could be substituted for vitamin A supplements.

The only side effect of taking too much beta-carotene is not dangerous: People who eat excessive amounts of foods high in beta-carotene may develop a yellowish-orange discoloration of the skin called *hypercarotenodermia*. This condition disappears within weeks once beta-carotene intake is reduced, and should not have any lasting or permanent adverse effects.

OPTIMAL DAILY ALLOWANCES

The important idea to keep in mind for vitamin A intake is that you want to derive maximum benefits from this important nutrient, while minimizing the risk of toxicity. The first and most important step is to keep your intake of preformed vitamin A well below the level that can produce adverse effects. The Optimal Daily Allowance of preformed vitamin A is 1,000 micrograms of RE (retinol equivalents), or 5,000 international units (IU); you should not exceed this amount.

It is possible to achieve the ODA of vitamin A by consuming mixed carotenoids. I recommend that you take in 6 to 15 milligrams of mixed carotenoids daily in addition to the preformed vitamin A. (Note that 15 milligrams is equivalent to about 25,000 international units of vitamin A.) The carotenoids have a similar biological activity to preformed vitamin A, but they do not appear to cause toxicity. Plus, you will benefit from their extra antioxidant activity.

Finally, if you take a supplement of mixed carotenoids to bring you up to the ODA of carotenoids, you do not need any supplemental vitamin A.

Food Sources

Vitamin A occurs naturally only in foods of animal origin, such as dairy products, including milk, cheese, butter, and ice cream; egg yolks; fish and fish oils; and liver and other organ meats. Some food products, including margarine and certain breakfast cereals, are fortified with vitamin A. Milk, already a known source of vitamin A, is sometimes fortified with extra amounts of the nutrient.

Much of the vitamin A that comes from dietary sources is supplied indirectly by the carotenoids, including beta-carotene, which are found in many vegetables and fruits. Good sources of the carotenoids include yellow and orange vegetables, such as carrots, sweet potatoes, and pumpkins; green leafy vegetables, including spinach, broccoli, collard greens, turnip greens, and peppers; and yellow and orange fruits like papayas, oranges, apricots, peaches, and cantaloupes.

While nutrient tables—such as those found in this book—are useful guides in determining the vitamin A and beta-carotene contents of many foods, they are not always helpful for precise assessments. The amounts of vitamin A in foods from animal sources can vary, particularly in meat and dairy products, depending on the diet of the animal that the product came from. The carotenoid content can vary, too, depending on growing conditions for the fruits and vegetables. Additionally, a great deal of the vitamin A and beta-carotene content of foods can be lost when the foods are processed and stored, and these nutrients can also be destroyed by exposure to heat and light.

Are You Maximizing Your Vitamin A Intake?

By eating plenty of the right fruits and vegetables, it is possible to take in 1,000 micrograms of vitamin A and 6 to 15 milligrams of carotenoids each day through diet alone. However, scientific research suggests that most people don't take in the amounts of these nutrients that they need to achieve optimal health.

The Second National Health and Nutrition Examination Survey (NHANES) revealed that only 20 percent of the individuals surveyed ate any fruits or vegetables rich in beta-carotene on the day they were questioned. According to the government's Continuing Survey of Food Intakes by Individuals for 1994, women consumed an average of 953 micrograms of RE of vitamin A per day, which is above the RDA of 800 micrograms for adult women. However, on average, the women surveyed consumed only 0.5 milligrams of carotenoids each day. (Statistics for men are not available.) This intake is far below the 6 milligrams of beta-carotene needed to meet the guidelines established by the U.S. Department of Agriculture (USDA) and the National Cancer Institute (NCI)—and far below the higher end of the ODA range. Statistically speaking it seems that many people could benefit greatly from supplementation. Where do you stand?

You can use the information in Tables 5.1 and 5.2 to determine your average daily intake of vitamin A and the carotenoids. The foods and beverages included in these two tables are arranged according to the percentage of the Optimal Daily Allowance of vitamin A and carotenoids they contain. Remember, the ODA of vitamin A is 100 micrograms of RE; the ODA of carotenoids is 6 to 15 milligrams. For this self-test, we will use the ODA of vitamin A.

Start by keeping a food diary for at least three to four days; the longer you keep the diary, the more accurate your calculations will be. Write down everything you eat and drink, as well as the estimated serving size, and refer to the tables on pages 63 and 64 to determine the percentage of the ODA that each food or beverage provides. At the end of the day, add up all of the percentages to see if you've reached 100 percent for the day.

If you find that, on average, you do not take in 100 percent of your ODAs for vitamin A and carotenoids, then you may decide that you want to take vitamin supplements for optimal health. But how much of these nutrients do you need to take to reach your ODAs for these nutrients? Here's an example of how to perform this calculation: Let's say you discover that you're getting 50 per-

Table 5.1. Percent of Vitamin A ODA in Common Foods and Beverages

Food	Serving Size	Food	Serving Size
5 Percent		Prunes, dried	10 prunes
American cheese	1 ounce	Ricotta cheese, part-skim	½ cup
Asparagus, boiled	6 spears	Swordfish	3 ounces
Avocado	½ medium	Tomato	1 medium
Blue cheese	1 ounce	Tomato juice, canned	6 ounces
Brussels sprouts	4 sprouts	**20 Percent**	
Camembert	1 ounce	Apricots	3 medium
Cheddar cheese	1 ounce	Beef soup, chunky	1 cup
Colby cheese	1 ounce	Clams	4 large or 9 small
Egg	1 large		
Guava	1 medium	Marinara sauce	1 cup
Herring	3 ounces	Mustard greens, boiled	½ cup
Ice milk, vanilla	1 cup	Swiss chard, boiled	½ cup
Lobster	3 ounces	Turnip greens, boiled	½ cup
Mozzarella cheese	1 ounce	**30 Percent**	
Muenster cheese	1 ounce	Beet greens, boiled	½ cup
Provolone cheese	1 ounce	Bran Flakes cereal	1 ounce
Sardines, canned in oil	2 sardines	Corn Flakes cereal	1 ounce
Swiss cheese	1 ounce	Cream of Wheat, instant	1 packet
Tangerine	1 medium	Kale, boiled	½ cup
10 Percent		Manhattan clam chowder	1 cup
Broccoli, boiled	½ cup		
Butter	1 tablespoon	Oatmeal, instant	1 packet
Chicken soup, chunky	1 cup	Raisin Bran cereal	1 ounce
Cream cheese	1 ounce	**50 Percent**	
Halibut	3 ounces	Cantaloupe pieces	1 cup
Ice cream, vanilla	1 cup	Vegetable soup, chunky	1 cup
Mackerel	3 ounces	**60 Percent**	
Milk, 1%	1 cup	Hubbard squash, baked	½ cup
Nectarine	1 medium	**70 Percent**	
Parsley	½ cup	Butternut squash, boiled	½ cup

Food	Serving Size	Food	Serving Size
80 Percent		Carrot juice, canned	6 ounces
Mango	1 medium	Chicken liver, simmered	3½ ounces
100 Percent or More		Product 19 cereal	1 ounce
Beef liver, braised	3½ ounces	Sweet potato, baked	1 ounce
Carrot	1 medium	Total cereal	1 ounce

Table 5.2. Percent of Carotenoids ODA in Common Foods and Beverages

Food	Serving Size	Food	Serving Size
5 Percent		Spinach	½ cup
Beet greens, boiled	1 cup	Tomato juice, canned	1 cup
Broccoli, cooked	½ cup	**20 Percent**	
Celery	1 cup	Apricot, dried	7 halves
Guava	½ cup	Fennel leaves	1 cup
Ketchup	1 tablespoon	Kale	1 cup
Leek	1 cup	Pepper, red	1 cup
Mango	½ mango	Sweet potato, baked	⅓ cup
Romaine lettuce	1 cup	Winter squash,	
Scallion	1 cup	cooked	½ cup
Swiss chard	1 cup	**30 Percent**	
Tomato	1 cup	Cantaloupe	1 cup
Tomato paste, canned	2 ounces	Spinach	½ cup
Tomato sauce, canned	½ cup	**40 Percent**	
10 Percent		Carrots	½ cup
Apricot, canned	½ cup	Chicory leaf	½ cup
Cress leaf	½ cup	**60 Percent**	
Grapefruit, pink	½ medium	Carrots, canned	½ cup
Mustard greens	1 cup	Collard greens, boiled	1 cup
Peach, dried	1 whole	**100 Percent or More**	
Pumpkin	½ cup	Apricots	4 medium

cent (0.50) of your target intake through diet alone. Multiply 0.50 by 1,000 micrograms (the ODA of vitamin A), and you'll find that you're consuming 500 micrograms of vitamin A in your diet. To make up the difference, then, you should take in 500 micrograms daily of vitamin A in supplement form.

Keep in mind that if you take carotenoid supplements to reach your ODA, you don't need supplemental vitamin A. You can take both, but only the carotenoids are necessary.

RECOMMENDATIONS

When it comes to nutrition, there's a lot of important information to remember—so it helps to have what you need to know right at your fingertips. The most critical facts about vitamin A are summarized below.

What are the Optimal Daily Allowances of vitamin A and the carotenoids?
The ODA of vitamin A is 1,000 micrograms of RE, equivalent to 5,000 international units; of carotenoids, it is 6 to 15 milligrams. Remember that if you take a mixed-carotenoid supplement to reach your Optimal Daily Allowance, you don't need to take supplemental vitamin A.

What circumstances might affect the amounts of vitamin A and carotenoids you need to take in each day?
Some lifestyle or health factors can affect the amount of vitamin A and beta-carotene you consume or decrease the amount that your body is able to absorb and use. You'll have to be particularly conscientious about taking in the ODAs of vitamin A and beta-carotene if:

- You have a chronic liver disease, such as hepatitis, cirrhosis, or liver cancer.

- You suffer from chronic diarrhea.

- You take certain medications, including cholesterol-lowering drugs and mineral oil.

- You use oral contraceptives.

- You drink large amounts of alcohol.

- You smoke cigarettes.

- You are under a great deal of physical or emotional stress.

- You are pregnant or breast-feeding.

Is it possible to consume the optimal amount of vitamin A and mixed carotenoids through diet alone?
It is indeed possible to reach the ODA of vitamin A and the carotenoids by eating plenty of the right fruits and vegetables, including yellow and orange vegetables, such as carrots and sweet potatoes; green leafy vegetables, including broccoli, spinach, and collard greens; and yellow and orange fruits like papayas, oranges, and cantaloupes. However, studies suggest that many people fail to take in the ODA of vitamin A and the carotenoids, and would probably benefit from supplementation.

Chapter 6

Vitamin D

Vitamin D is not like other vitamins. In fact, this nutrient does not meet the classic definition of a vitamin because the body can make all it needs with the help of the sun's ultraviolet rays. However, people who do not get adequate sunlight throughout the year may need to take in vitamin D through dietary sources. Elderly people may also need dietary vitamin D because their bodies cannot manufacture enough of the nutrient.

Vitamin D is actually an umbrella term that covers a family of fat-soluble compounds. D vitamins, or *calciferols*, come in many forms, but only two—D_2 and D_3—are important in the human body. Vitamin D_2, also known as *ergocalciferol*, is produced when a substance in plants called ergosterol is irradiated. This form of the vitamin is usually found in vitamin supplements. Also, some dietary sources, including milk, are fortified with vitamin D_2. Vitamin D_3, also called *cholecalciferol*, is a natural form of vitamin D that is made when the skin is exposed to sunlight. This type of vitamin D is contained in foods from animal sources.

FUNCTIONS IN THE BODY

Vitamin D is an essential nutrient for maintaining bone density. This is news to many people, because the emphasis always falls much more heavily on the role of calcium in promoting healthy bones. The fact is, without vitamin D, the body would not be able to use calcium to build bones. Vitamin D enhances the absorption of the bone-building minerals, such as calcium and phosphorus, in the intestine. It also regulates the amounts of calcium and phosphorous in the blood.

In its active form, vitamin D is involved in the growth and maturation of cells essential to healthy immune system function. A lesser known function of vitamin D is its role in stimulating the production of insulin, a hormone produced by the pancreas. In the case of a vitamin D deficiency, the body may not be able to manufacture enough insulin to handle simple sugars (glucose). This can contribute to the development of diabetes.

HEALTH BENEFITS

Some of the strongest evidence pointing to vitamin D's benefits in the body concerns the nutrient's ability to protect against osteoporosis—the thinning of the bones—and bone fractures that can result from this condition. By maintaining sufficient blood levels of calcium, vitamin D promotes bone mineralization, thereby strengthening the bones.

Osteoporosis is a common and sometimes crippling disorder in which the bones become porous and fragile. This degenerative condition primarily affects women, and statistics show that half of all women between the ages of forty-five and seventy show some signs of osteoporosis. While calcium supplementation is an important defense against osteoporosis, most doctors urge older female patients to take in adequate amounts of vitamin D in addition to calcium. The results of several studies of vitamin D's effects on osteoporosis have convinced physicians to make this recommendation.

In 1987, researchers in Amsterdam, the Netherlands, evaluated the role of vitamin D supplements in preventing hip fractures in both men and women. The researchers measured blood levels of vitamin D in 125 older men and women with hip fractures, and in 74 men and women without fractures. Vitamin D levels were notably lower in the individuals who had hip fractures.

A study conducted in 1991 at Tufts University in Boston, Massachusetts, also provided supporting evidence for the valuable role vitamin D plays in preventing osteoporosis. In this study, postmenopausal women took either 400 international units daily of supplemental vitamin D or a placebo, with no active ingredients.

Are You at Risk of Vitamin D Deficiency?

How do you know if you're at risk of vitamin D deficiency? Take a moment to review the questions below. If you answer yes to any of these questions, you have an above-average risk of developing a deficiency.

❏ *Do you spend most of your time indoors, away from natural sunlight?* Adequate sunlight is essential to the body's manufacture of vitamin D. With limited sun exposure, only a minimal amount of vitamin D is produced by the skin. If this is the case, you may have to rely entirely on dietary sources to meet your needs for this important nutrient.

❏ *Do you have kidney or liver disease?* While vitamin D can be manufactured in the skin, the nutrient has to be chemically modified by the kidneys and liver before it can be used by the body. If the function of either of these organs is impaired, then the body cannot effectively use natural vitamin D.

❏ *Do you take cholesterol-lowering medications?* Cholesterol-lowering agents—including cholestyramine and colestipol—can diminish the body's ability to absorb vitamin D.

❏ *Do you take anticonvulsant medications?* Drugs such as phenytoin, phenobarbital, and primidone convert vitamin D to an inactive form.

❏ *Do you use mineral oil as a laxative?* The use of mineral oil may cause vitamin D deficiency because fat-soluble vitamins dissolve in the indigestible oil and are excreted.

❏ *Do you drink large amounts of alcohol?* Alcohol appears to reduce blood levels of vitamin D and lowers absorption of the nutrient by the intestines. Also, alcoholics tend to substitute alcohol—which has no real nutritional value—for nutrient-dense foods, so they may not take in adequate amounts of vitamin D and other nutrients.

❏ *Are you an older person?* The production of vitamin D by the skin occurs at a reduced rate as the years pass. Studies of older people—particularly older women—show that as many as 75 percent have an increased risk of vitamin D deficiency.

The women involved in the study also took 377 milligrams of supplemental calcium per day. Every six months, the researchers measured bone density in these participants. After one year, the women treated with vitamin D showed modest increases in bone mineral density; the women who took the placebo showed no significant effects. The benefits were most noticeable during the last six months of the study—from December/January through June/July—when the body's own production of vitamin D tends to be lower because of decreased sun exposure.

Further research, conducted in 1992 in Lyon, France, looked at the effects of calcium and vitamin D supplementation on bone density in 3,270 elderly women. The participants in this study took either 800 international units of vitamin D plus 1.2 grams of supplemental calcium per day, or two placebo pills. After eighteen months, the women who had taken vitamin D and calcium had suffered 43 percent fewer hip fractures and 32 percent fewer other nonvertebral fractures—such as those of the wrist, forearm, humerus, and pelvis—than those who had taken the placebo pills.

DEFICIENCY SYMPTOMS

Two common disorders caused by vitamin D deficiency are *rickets* and *osteomalacia*. Rickets is primarily a childhood disease. It is the most widely acknowledged disorder associated with vitamin D deficiency.

Without sufficient vitamin D, bones cannot grow strong and healthy because calcium is not used effectively. The bones of people who have rickets soften and become so pliable that they bend, which can cause skeletal problems such as knock-knees, bowlegs, and pelvic and spine deformities. This deficiency disease can also cause the breastbone to become misshapen so that the chest is sunken, which can lead to problems with the lungs and breathing difficulties.

Rickets is rare in most parts of the world today, thanks largely to the availability of foods rich in vitamin D, either naturally or through fortification. Children who are breast-fed for a long time without vitamin D supplementation do have an increased chance of developing this disease, however. Today, rickets occurs most often in children under three years of age.

When There's Too Little Sun

Because your skin can manufacture vitamin D when it is exposed to sunlight, you may not require any vitamin D in your diet. Don't ignore dietary vitamin D completely, however, without thinking about your particular situation. How much time do you spend in the sun? How much of your skin is actually exposed to the sun? Do any environmental conditions—smog, fog, sunscreen, or window glass—keep ultraviolet light from reaching your skin? These are important factors in determining whether or not your body can produce all the vitamin D it needs.

Additionally, remember that in older people, vitamin D is produced by the skin at about half the rate at which it's produced in younger people. Consequently, older individuals should be careful to include vitamin D-rich foods in their diets. Skin pigment is another important factor to consider; people with dark skin need more sun exposure than do people with light skin to produce the same amount of vitamin D. Also, people who live very far from the equator are exposed to less sunlight and therefore may not produce the vitamin as efficiently.

Osteomalacia is similar to rickets, and may occur in adults who are vitamin D deficient. This condition involves the same kind of softening of the bones; it is produced by inadequate calcification of the bones—in other words, by a lack of sufficient calcium in the bones. Left untreated, osteomalacia weakens the bones, making them more subject to fractures. It may also cause bowed legs.

TOXICITY SYMPTOMS

If too much vitamin D can be toxic in your body, you might wonder if too much time in the sun will cause your body to manufacture and store excess amounts of the vitamin. The simple answer is no. While overexposure to the sun will raise your risk of developing skin cancer, it won't cause toxic accumulations of vitamin D. When the body has produced enough of the nutrient, a feedback system automatically cuts back the manufacturing process.

What about vitamin D supplements? Excess vitamin D taken in

through supplements *can* be toxic. Remember, vitamin D is fat-soluble, so the body stores extra amounts in the fat tissues; the excess is not excreted quickly, as it is with water-soluble vitamins. Indeed, high levels of vitamin D can remain in the body for weeks—even months.

In infants, doses as low as 1,800 international units per day can be toxic. In adults, symptoms of toxicity generally don't appear until much higher intake levels are reached—generally about 50,000 international units daily. Because young children run a greater risk of developing symptoms of toxicity at lower levels than adults, be cautious about giving supplements to youngsters. Before you give your child vitamin D supplements, check with your pediatrician or family doctor. Some doctors do advise giving a supplement of up to 400 international units of vitamin D per day to breast-fed babies or babies fed formula that is not fortified with vitamin D. Pediatricians may also suggest supplements for older children—particularly those who don't drink milk.

Symptoms of toxicity include nausea, weakness, headache, and constipation, all of which can be treated successfully. A more serious complication associated with toxic levels of vitamin D is a condition known as *hypercalcemia*, which can lead to the formation of calcium deposits in the heart, blood vessels, and kidneys.

OPTIMAL DAILY ALLOWANCE

The Optimal Daily Allowance of vitamin D for men and women is 400 international units. Fewer foods are rich in vitamin D than in other vitamins and minerals, so you may need to take a vitamin D supplement to reach this ODA.

Although the risk of toxicity is relatively low from moderate doses of vitamin D, taking more than 400 international units per day is not recommended at this time.

Food Sources

The best sources of natural vitamin D include eggs; butter; oily fish, such as salmon, herring, and sardines; liver; and cod liver oil. Plant foods are *not* good sources of this nutrient. Green leafy vegetables, for example, contain only small amounts of vitamin D.

Most of our dietary vitamin D comes from foods that have been fortified. Cow's milk is usually fortified with vitamin D and is the primary source of this nutrient for children. Infant formula is also fortified with vitamin D. Other commonly fortified foods include margarine and ready-to-eat breakfast cereals.

Vitamin D is a remarkably stable nutrient, so little of it is lost due to cooking and storage.

Are You Maximizing Your Vitamin D Intake?

Although it is possible to consume 400 international units of vitamin D per day, many people fail to achieve this intake, primarily because there aren't many vitamin D-rich foods to choose from. One could easily reach the ODA by drinking three 8-ounce glasses of milk every day—which supplies about 300 international units— and then making up the difference by eating foods that contain even small amounts of vitamin D, and spending some time in the sun. However, researchers have found that the average woman takes in less than 100 international units daily, and the average man doesn't even get close to 100—proof that most adults don't drink three glasses of milk on any given day. Where do you stand?

You can use the information in Table 6.1 to determine your average daily intake of vitamin D. The foods and beverages included in this table are arranged according to the percentage of the Optimal Daily Allowance of vitamin D they contain. Start by keeping a food diary for at least three to four days; the longer you keep the diary, the more accurate your calculations will be. Write down everything you eat and drink, as well as the estimated serving size, and refer to the table on page 74 to determine the percentage of the ODA that each food or beverage provides. At the end of each day, add up all of the percentages to see if you've reached 100 percent for the day.

If you find that, on average, you do not take in 100 percent of your ODA for vitamin D, then you may decide that you want to take vitamin supplements for optimal health. But how much of this nutrient do you need to take to reach your ODA? Here's an example of how to perform this calculation: Let's say you discover that you're getting 60 percent (0.60) of your target intake through diet alone. Multiply 0.60 by 400 international units (the ODA of

Table 6.1. Percent of Vitamin D ODA in Common Foods and Beverages

Food	Serving Size	Food	Serving Size
10 Percent		**60 Percent**	
Egg	1 large	Sardines, canned	3 ounces
25 Percent		**100 Percent or More**	
Milk	1 cup	Cod liver oil	1 tablespoon
50 Percent		Herring, grilled	3 ounces
Tuna, canned in oil	3 ounces	Mackerel, fried	3 ounces

vitamin D), and you'll find that you are consuming 240 international units of vitamin D in your diet. To make up the difference, then, you should take in 160 international units of vitamin D in supplement form.

Because vitamin D is commonly sold in doses of 100, 200, or 400 international units, you may have some trouble finding a supplement that contains the exact amount you want. Try to get as close as you can to your supplemental needs without taking several pills or cutting the pills in half. In the example cited here, you can meet your needs by taking a supplement that contains 200 international units of vitamin D, which will be enough to help you reach your ODA without the risk of adverse effects.

RECOMMENDATIONS

When it comes to nutrition, there's a lot of important information to remember—so it helps to have what you need to know right at your fingertips. The most critical facts about vitamin D are summarized below.

What is the Optimal Daily Allowance of vitamin D?
The ODA of vitamin D for men and women is 400 international units. Taking more than this amount is not recommended.

What circumstances might affect the amount of vitamin D you need to take in each day?
Some lifestyle or health factors can affect the amount of vitamin D

you consume or decrease the amount that your body is able to absorb and use. You'll have to be particularly conscientious about taking in the ODA of vitamin D if:

- You spend most of your time indoors, away from natural light.

- You suffer from kidney or liver disease.

- You take certain medications, including cholesterol-lowering drugs, anitconvulsants, or mineral oil.

- You drink large amounts of alcohol.

- You are an older person.

Is it possible to consume the optimal amount of vitamin D through diet alone?
While it's possible to reach the ODA of vitamin D, it seems that many people fail to do so, partly because there are few vitamin D-rich foods. By drinking three 8-ounce glasses of milk each day—containing as much as 300 international units of vitamin D—you'll be well on your way to meeting the ODA. However, most adults don't drink much milk, and statistics show that women and men often fail to take in the daily allowance. Because sources of dietary vitamin D are not plentiful, supplementation is a wise idea.

Chapter 7

Vitamin E

Few nutrients have been the subject of as much discussion as vitamin E has in recent years. The most ardent proponents of the nutrient believe that it's nothing short of a magic pill that can do a little bit of everything, from enhancing sexual function to slowing the aging process. While it's doubtful that any nutrient—even a powerful antioxidant such as vitamin E—can cure every ill, a growing body of evidence shows that vitamin E does provide significant health benefits. The real challenge is to sort scientific fact from fiction in the wake of the commotion surrounding this popular nutrient.

Vitamin E actually consists of a group of fat-soluble compounds that fall into two different categories: the *tocopherols* and the *tocotrienols*. The tocopherols are the more active of the two groups. Of these, alpha-tocopherol is the most potent form, and this name is often used interchangeably with vitamin E. The beta-, gamma-, and delta-tocopherols differ slightly in chemical structure and generally have lower vitamin E activity.

FUNCTIONS IN THE BODY

Vitamin E is a potent antioxidant that protects cells against the effects of oxidation by neutralizing highly unstable molecules known as free radicals. As you will remember from Chapter 3, free radicals are formed when the body combines oxygen with macronutrients—carbohydrates, fats, and proteins—to produce energy. Free-radical formation is excessive in times of physical stress, such

The History of Vitamin E

In 1922, researchers stumbled upon a mysterious substance in lettuce and wheat germ that appeared to restore the reproductive function of rats. The scientists had been observing female rats that were placed on a restricted, nutrient-poor diet. Although these rats were able to conceive, the fetuses typically died before birth. When lettuce or wheat germ was added to their diets, however, normal reproduction resulted. The scientists could not identify the specific chemical substance in these foods, so they named it "Factor X."

Additional animal studies resulted in similar findings. For example, male rats fed a Factor X-deficient diet suffered reproductive abnormalities, including testicular atrophy. For a time, this elusive nutrient was called the "fertility vitamin." Finally, in 1936, vitamin E was isolated and named.

as during intense exercise, and also because of exposure to environmental pollution and radiation.

Vitamin E helps protect cells by inhibiting the oxidation of phospholipids, the fats contained in cell membranes that are highly susceptible to attack by free radicals. In fact, because vitamin E is fat-soluble, it functions most effectively in this type of environment. Working as an antioxidant, vitamin E protects the lungs against injury from air pollution, guards against free-radical damage throughout the body, and may impede the development of tumors. It also prevents the oxidative destruction of other nutrients, including vitamins A and C, as well as beta-carotene. And evidence suggests that vitamin E works synergistically with other antioxidants, such as vitamin C. This means that the two nutrients have a greater impact when they work together than when they work separately.

Research has shown that vitamin E may work as a preventive agent against certain degenerative diseases, including cancer and cardiovascular disease, and conditions such as cataracts.

HEALTH BENEFITS

The studies that have so far been conducted on the health benefits of vitamin E have produced some very impressive findings that point to the vitamin's protective effects against cancer, cardiovascular disease, and cataracts. Research has also shown that vitamin E can help boost immunity and may even be useful in the treatment of neurological disorders such as Parkinson's disease.

Cancer

A growing body of research indicates that vitamin E can provide protection against several types of cancer, including cancers of the mouth, lungs, cervix, and breast. In a study conducted in Finland over a period of eight years, researchers compared blood levels of the alpha-tocopherol form of vitamin E in 36,265 adults. The investigators concluded that individuals with low blood levels of alpha-tocopherol were 1.5 times more likely to develop cancer than people with higher blood levels of the nutrient. And while skeptics may choose to focus on research that has not demonstrated the protective effects of vitamin E against cancer, some of these reports have even found that individuals who are free of the disease have higher vitamin E levels than do individuals with the disease—although the differences may not be great enough to have what researchers call "statistical significance."

Cancers of the Mouth and Throat

In 1992, researchers at the National Cancer Institute compared the use of vitamin supplements by 1,114 patients with oral and pharyngeal (throat) cancers with the use of supplements by 1,268 cancer-free individuals. This study indicated that use of vitamin E supplements reduces an individual's chance of developing these cancers. People who used supplements regularly for six or more months were only half as likely to develop these cancers as people who had never taken supplemental vitamin E regularly.

Lung Cancer

A study of vitamin E's effects on lung cancer, conducted at Louisiana State University Medical Center, involved fifty-nine people who had recently been diagnosed as having lung cancer. Researchers measured vitamin blood levels—including blood levels of vitamin E—of the participants, and then compared these measurements with those of a similar number of cancer-free individuals. The results, published in 1990, showed that the individuals with lung cancer had significantly lower blood levels of vitamin E.

In another study, starting in 1974, researchers at the Johns Hopkins School of Hygiene and Public Health drew and froze blood samples from more than 25,000 people. During the span of the study, ninety-nine of the participants developed lung cancer. Researchers found that the average vitamin E levels were significantly lower in the blood samples from individuals with cancer, when compared with blood levels of vitamin E in samples from 196 cancer-free individuals. In a report published in 1991, the researchers concluded that participants with blood levels of vitamin E ranking in the lowest 20 percent had a two-and-a-half times greater risk of developing lung cancer than did participants whose levels were in the highest 20 percent.

Scientists in Finland conducted a study to investigate the effects of antioxidant nutrients on the risk of lung cancer in 4,538 men. Beginning in the early 1970s, the researchers performed initial screening tests and took careful dietary histories of the participants, and then closely monitored the health of these men over the course of twenty years. During this period, 117 participants were diagnosed with lung cancer. The findings of this study, published in 1991, showed that nonsmokers who consumed the least amounts of vitamin E were three times more likely to develop lung cancer, compared with individuals who took the highest doses. Vitamin E did not appear to protect smokers against cancer.

There is one other study that deserves our attention here. In 1994, research conducted in the United States and in Finland investigated the possible health benefits of vitamin E and beta-carotene for long-term smokers. As a result of this widely-publicized study, researchers came to the unexpected conclusion that neither vitamin E nor beta-carotene protected smokers from lung cancer. (See page 54 for more details about this study.) However, the research did show that fewer cases of prostate cancer occurred in men who supplemented with vitamin E.

It's important to note that the dose used in the U.S./Finnish study was less than the Optimal Daily Allowance of vitamin E and less than the amount contained in most supplements. In addition, the fact that all of the participants in this study were cigarette smokers is a reminder that taking vitamins cannot remove all of the risks associated with unhealthful behaviors.

Cervical Cancer

Adequate intake of vitamin E also appears to be important for protection against cervical cancer. This was demonstrated in a study conducted in the Seattle area of Washington, in which 189 women diagnosed with cervical cancer and 227 cancer-free women filled out dietary questionnaires about their intakes of vitamins A, C, and E, folic acid, and other nutrients. In 1989, the researchers published their report, stating that high intake of vitamin E reduced the risk of developing cervical cancer. The results of the study showed that women in the top 25 percent for vitamin E intake were only one-third as likely to have cancer as those in the bottom 25 percent.

Another study that highlighted vitamin E's effectiveness in preventing cervical cancer was conducted at the Albert Einstein College of Medicine in New York. At the start of this study, researchers collected blood samples from 116 women. Of these participants, thirty-six had no cervical disease, while the other eighty had abnormal Pap smears, although the lesions that were detected had not yet progressed to cancer. In their evaluations of the antioxidant levels in these blood samples, the researchers found that blood levels of vitamin E were significantly lower in women with cervical dysplasia (characterized by irregular cells that may develop into cancer) than were blood levels in women whose Pap smears were normal. The relationship was graded; women with the most severe lesions had the lowest blood levels of vitamin E.

Breast Cancer

In a 1984 study conducted at the Medical College of St. Bartholomew's Hospital in London, England, researchers drew blood samples from more than five thousand women, and then monitored the women for the development of breast cancer. Over the next several years, thirty-nine of the women developed breast cancer. When their blood levels of antioxidants were compared with the levels of seventy-eight women who had remained free of cancer, the results showed that low levels of vitamin E were associated with a much higher risk of cancer. In fact, women with the lowest vitamin E levels were five times more likely to develop cancer than were women with the highest levels.

Prostate Cancer

Vitamin E also appears to offer protection against prostate cancer. A study conducted in Finland evaluated the benefits of vitamin E for 29,133 male smokers, ranging in age from fifty to sixty-nine years old. About half of the participants supplemented with 50 milligrams of alpha-tocopherol a day for a period of five to eight years, while the rest of the participants took a placebo, with no active ingredients. The results of this research, published in 1998 in the *Journal of the National Cancer Institute,* showed that the rate of prostate cancer was 41 percent lower among men who took vitamin E, when compared with the group taking the placebo.

Cardiovascular Disease

Vitamin E has become known for its possible protective effects against cardiovascular disease. Researchers suspect that the vitamin helps protect against atherosclerosis, or hardening of the arteries, by preventing the oxidation of low-density lipoprotein (LDL) cholesterol. LDL is often called the "bad" cholesterol because it causes the buildup of fatty deposits along the inside walls of the arteries.

The Health Professionals Study, which began in 1986, involved nearly 40,000 male health workers, ranging in age from forty to seventy-five years old. All of these participants were free of heart disease. At the start of the study, the men filled out dietary questionnaires that asked for information about their intake of a variety of nutrients, including antioxidants such as vitamin E. Over the next four years, 667 of the participants were diagnosed as having coronary heart disease, which includes heart attacks or heart conditions requiring angioplasty. After analyzing these cases, the researchers concluded that men in the top fifth of the group for vitamin E consumption had a 41 percent lower risk of coronary disease than men in the bottom fifth. According to the study, published in 1993, men who consumed 100 to 249 international units per day were best protected; men who took 100 international units or more of vitamin E supplements for at least two years had a 37-percent lower risk of heart disease than those who did not take supplements.

The Nurses' Health Study, which began in 1980, looked at the effects of antioxidants on heart disease in women. This study involved more than 87,000 female nurses, ranging in age from thirty-four to fifty-nine years old and all free of heart disease. The participants were asked to fill out dietary questionnaires to determine their intakes of a variety of nutrients, including vitamin E, and then their health was monitored over the course of several years. Within eight years of filling out their questionnaires, 552 of these women were diagnosed with coronary heart disease. In 1993, the researchers reported that the women with the highest vitamin E intake—due to supplementation—were 34 percent less likely to develop major heart disease than women with the lowest intake of the vitamin. The risk of coronary disease in women who had taken vitamin E supplements for two years or more was 41 percent lower than the risk in unsupplemented participants.

At the University of Southern California School of Medicine, investigators studied the effects of supplementation with vitamins C and E upon the progression of coronary artery disease, which is characterized by the buildup of plaque in the arteries that supply oxygen and nutrients to the heart. More than 150 men, forty to fifty-nine years old, participated in the study; all had previously undergone coronary bypass surgery. In 1995, the researchers revealed that, overall, men who took 100 international units or more per day of vitamin E experienced less progression of their heart disease, compared with men who took less than 100 international units. These improvements were particularly evident in a group of men who were also taking a combination of colestipol and niacin to lower cholesterol.

According to a study published in *JAMA (The Journal of the American Medical Association)* in 1996, vitamin E may have other benefits relative to cardiovascular disease. Specifically, it seems that the nutrient can help reduce the incidence of a severe type of chest pain called angina. The National Public Health Institute in Finland, along with the United States National Cancer Institute, conducted research to evaluate the effects of vitamin E and beta-carotene on angina in 22,000 male smokers with no known coronary heart disease. The participants in the study were divided into four groups: One group of men took 50 milligrams daily of vitamin E; another group supplemented with 20 milligrams per day of beta-carotene; a third group supplemented with both nutrients; and the rest of the men took a placebo. After nearly five years, the men who took only vitamin E supplements were 9 percent less likely to experience angina than those who did not take vitamin E.

In 1986, researchers at the University of Minnesota School of Public Health and other institutions conducted a study to investigate the risk of coronary heart disease (CHD) in postmenopausal women. These researchers determined the vitamin A, C, and E intakes of more than 34,000 CHD-free women, ranging in age from fifty-five to sixty-nine years old. Then, the health of the participants was monitored over the course of seven years. The report, which was published in 1996, showed that women who consumed more vitamin E in their diets were less likely to die of CHD than women whose vitamin E intakes were lower. In fact, the women whose diets contained the largest amounts of vitamin E had a 62 percent lower risk of dying from heart disease than women with the lowest vitamin E intakes from dietary sources—a very significant difference.

Immune System Function

The immune system is responsible for defending against invading bacteria, viruses, and other disease-causing agents that might otherwise cause illnesses and infections in the body. Studies have shown that vitamin E deficiency can undermine the body's resistance to disease, and thus may increase the vulnerability to a variety of disorders, such as infections in older people, as well as cancers associated with increasing age.

A 1990 study conducted at Tufts University in Boston evaluated the effect of vitamin E on immunity in healthy men and women aged sixty and older. The thirty-two participants in this study were given either 800 international units of vitamin E every day for a month or a placebo. When the month was up, the researchers found that several measures of immune function had improved in the group that supplemented with vitamin E; subjects taking the placebo did not experience these positive changes.

Cataracts

Cataracts are one of the leading causes of blindness among older people. Some research indicates that vitamin E, taken in conjunction with vitamin C and carotenoids, may effectively delay the development of cataracts. These antioxidants work by interfering with the oxidation of proteins in the lens of the eye, a process that is believed to cause the clouding and opacity of the lens that occurs with cataracts.

In a study conducted in 1991 at the University of Western Ontario, Canada, investigators examined the effects of vitamin supplements on the development of cataracts in 350 men and women. The results showed that people with cataracts were 44 percent less likely to have taken vitamin E supplements than people without cataracts.

The correlation between blood levels of antioxidants and the development of cataracts was also studied in Finland in 1992. Researchers measured antioxidant levels in forty-seven men and women with cataracts and in ninety-four individuals without cataracts, and found that low levels of vitamin E and beta-carotene were linked to an increased risk of developing cataracts. More specifically, individuals in the lowest one-third of the group for vitamin E levels had a 90-percent greater chance of having cataracts than participants in the highest two-thirds.

Parkinson's Disease

Parkinson's disease is a degenerative disorder that affects the nerve centers in the brain, resulting in symptoms such as muscular rigidity, tremors, and impaired speech. Many experts believe that the cells are damaged and destroyed by toxins—such as free radicals—within the body. If this is true, then vitamin E's antioxidant powers may help slow or even halt the progression of this disease.

In a small study conducted at Columbia University's College of Physicians and Surgeons in New York, patients in the early stages of Parkinson's disease were given large doses of two antioxidants—3,200 milligrams daily of vitamin E and 3,000 milligrams daily of vitamin C. Doctors hoped that these nutrients might slow the progression of Parkinson's in the participants. According to the results, published in 1991, that's precisely what happened. Individuals taking the antioxidants were able to remain medication-free for extended periods of time; because their illness progressed more slowly, these patients were able to postpone starting treatment with a drug called levadopa for a full two-and-a-half years. However, a larger study using only vitamin E, taken in doses of 2,000 international units per day, failed to produce the same positive results.

Alzheimer's Disease

Alzheimer's disease is a degenerative condition characterized by physiological changes in the brain that cause the decline of cognitive and behavioral abilities. Eventually, the disease destroys memory, judgment, language, reasoning, and orientation. While scientists are still uncertain about the causes of Alzheimer's, some speculate that vitamin E's ability to combat free radicals could help prevent some of the nerve cell damage associated with this disease.

In 1997, researchers at Columbia University's College of Physicians and Surgeons studied the effects of vitamin E on the progression of Alzheimer's disease in several hundred men and women. One group of participants took 2,000 international units of vitamin E every day for two years, while a second group took a placebo. During the course of the study, the severity of the disease in these participants was monitored using a variety of endpoints, including: the need to be institutionalized; the loss of self-care skills, such as dressing, bathing, and using the toilet independently; the development of severe dementia, including total disorientation and even hallucinations; and, eventually, death. The research showed that treatment with vitamin E significantly slowed the progression of disease. On average, the men and women taking the placebo reached these disease endpoints 230 days sooner than individuals taking vitamin E.

DEFICIENCY SYMPTOMS

Severe vitamin E deficiencies are rare in the United States because vitamin E is common in most diets. Plus, reserves of this nutrient are stored in the tissues of the body, so one would have to consume low levels of vitamin E for months or even years for deficiency symptoms to develop.

When vitamin E deficiency does develop, it can impair a number of body functions, including those involved with the reproductive and nervous systems, and may also damage muscle tissues. Some of the most common symptoms are loss of appetite; anemia, due to loss of red blood cells from oxidative damage; mild gastrointestinal distress, such as nausea; eye problems, including cataracts and disorders of the retina; and impairment of the reproductive system, including testicular deterioration, decreased fertility, and an increased chance of spontaneous abortion (miscarriage). People who are deficient in vitamin E may also have difficulty walking, since free radicals can damage the cerebellum and brain stem in the absence of adequate levels of antioxidants.

TOXICITY SYMPTOMS

Vitamin E has been proven safe and virtually free of adverse effects when taken in doses of up to 800 international units (IU) daily. Indeed, in many trials, 3,200 milligrams—about 5,000 international units—per day have caused relatively few side effects.

However, occasional adverse reactions have been reported at extremely high doses. Symptoms include fatigue; nausea; headaches and double vision; weak muscles; breast tenderness in women; intestinal cramps and diarrhea; and emotional disturbances, such as depression, fatigue, and mood swings. Vitamin E can also interfere with the potency of anticoagulants, medications prescribed most often to prevent blood clotting in patients with heart disease. To avoid putting yourself at risk, stay within the vitamin E ODA range recommended on page 88. Intakes within this range have been proven safe for all adult men and women.

OPTIMAL DAILY ALLOWANCE

The amount of vitamin E that you need each day depends on your body size and the amount of polyunsaturated fats you consume. Vitamin E protects polyunsaturated fats in body tissues against oxidation. Thus, the more polyunsaturates in your diet, the greater

Are You at Risk of Vitamin E Deficiency?

How do you know if you're at risk of vitamin E deficiency? Take a moment to review the questions below. If you answer yes to any of these questions, you have an above-average risk of developing a deficiency.

❏ *Do you have one of the following chronic disorders: cystic fibrosis, pancreatitis, biliary cirrhosis, or Crohn's disease?* All of these conditions can interfere with the absorption of fat from the intestines, and so may result in vitamin E deficiency. In general, fat malabsorption must persist for five to ten years before deficiency symptoms develop.

❏ *Do you take cholesterol-lowering medications?* Cholesterol-lowering agents—including cholestyramine and colestipol—can diminish the body's ability to absorb vitamin E.

❏ *Do you use mineral oil as a laxative?* The use of mineral oil may cause vitamin E deficiency because fat-soluble vitamins dissolve in the indigestible oil and are excreted.

❏ *Do you smoke cigarettes?* Cigarette smoke causes oxidative damage to the body's healthy cells and tissues. People who smoke need greater amounts of antioxidants such as vitamin E to neutralize harmful free radicals.

your need for vitamin E. Because of these individual differences, it's difficult to determine a single intake level that's optimal for everyone.

Severe vitamin E deficiency is rare in the United States, so the primary consideration in determining your intake should be based on the amount you need for optimal health. High intakes can reduce the risk of chronic diseases and boost immune-system function, among other things.

The ODA of vitamin E ranges from 100 to 400 international units. The higher levels are appropriate for anyone with an increased risk of atherosclerosis and coronary heart disease, and for people who are at an above-average risk of deficiency.

❏ *Are you exposed to environmental pollution?* The body requires extra amounts of vitamin E and other antioxidants to protect against the free-radical damage that results from exposure to environmental pollutants.

❏ *Is your diet high in polyunsaturated fatty acids (PUFAs)?* PUFAs—found in corn, safflower, and sunflower oils—should be naturally high in vitamin E, which protects unsaturated fats against oxidation. Unfortunately, commercially processed oils generally contain little vitamin E, so the more of these oils you consume, the more vitamin E you need to prevent oxidation.

❏ *Are you on a low-fat or low-calorie diet to lose weight?* Individuals who reduce fat and calorie intake may not consume enough vitamin E each day.

❏ *Are you pregnant or breast-feeding?* Pregnancy is a time of increased nutritional needs because the growth of a new person requires every known nutrient. The National Research Council recommends a 25 percent increase in the RDA of vitamin E. Women who are breast-feeding should increase their vitamin E intake even more to compensate for the amount contained in breast milk. The ODA of vitamin E is more than adequate to meet the increased needs of women who are pregnant or breast-feeding.

Food Sources

Vitamin E is found in both animal and plant products. As a rule, plant products contain more vitamin E than do animal products. In addition, meats from animals that have diets high in fat may also be good sources of vitamin E, but because of their high fat content, it's better to get your vitamin E from plant sources.

What are the best sources of vitamin E? Vegetable oils—sunflower, soybean, corn, safflower, wheat-germ, and cottonseed oils —are all particularly rich in vitamin E, but the distribution of vitamin E compounds differs from one type of oil to another. For example, while the vitamin E content of safflower oil is 90 percent alpha-tocopherol—the most biologically active of the vitamin E compounds—corn oil has just 10 percent alpha-tocopherol. Other good sources of vitamin E are green leafy vegetables, liver, whole grains, wheat germ, butter, margarine, egg yolk, and nuts.

Cooking foods can deplete their vitamin E content. Also, cooking for long periods of time at high temperatures can destroy the vitamin E in oils.

Are You Maximizing Your Vitamin E Intake?

Practically speaking, it's almost impossible to reach the Optimal Daily Allowance of vitamin E from dietary sources alone. Therefore, almost everybody will benefit from vitamin E supplementation.

You can use the information in Table 7.1 to determine your average daily intake of vitamin A and the carotenoids. The foods and beverages included in this table are arranged according to the percentage of the Optimal Daily Allowance of vitamin E they contain. Remember, the ODA of vitamin E ranges from 100 to 400 international units. For this self-test, we'll use 100 international units.

Start by keeping a food diary for at least three to four days; the longer you keep the diary, the more accurate your calculations will be. Write down everything you eat and drink, as well as the estimated serving size, and refer to the table on page 91 to determine the percentage of the ODA that each food or beverage provides. At the end of each day, add up all of the percentages to see if you've reached 100 percent for the day. (If your optimal dose falls elsewhere in our recommended range, take that into account when calculating percentages.)

If you find that, on average, you do not take in 100 percent of your ODA for vitamin E, then you may decide that you want to take vitamin supplements for optimal health. But how much of these nutrients do you need to take to reach your ODA? Here's an example of how to perform this calculation: Let's say you discover that you're getting 20 percent (0.20) of your intake target through diet alone. Multiply 20 percent by 100 international units (the ODA of vitamin E), and you'll find that you're consuming 20 international units of vitamin E in your diet. To make up the difference, then, you should take in 80 international units of vitamin E in supplement form.

Because vitamin E is commonly sold in doses of 100 international units or more, you may have some trouble finding a supplement that contains the exact amount you need. Try to come as close as you can to your target intake without cutting up tablets to make the dose come out even. In the case just described, for example, you would probably need to go a little higher than 80 international units, and take a tablet that contains 100 international units, which will more than meet your optimal requirements without posing any risks to your health.

RECOMMENDATIONS

When it comes to nutrition, there's a lot of important information to remember—so it helps to have what you need to know right at your fingertips. The most critical facts about vitamin E are summarized below.

What is the Optimal Daily Allowance of vitamin E?
The ODA of vitamin E for men and women is 100 to 400 international units. This is several times higher than the RDA, since scientific evidence has shown that higher intakes of this nutrient can reduce the risk of chronic diseases and boost immune-system function.

Table 7.1. Percent of Vitamin E ODA in Common Foods and Beverages

Food	Serving Size	Food	Serving Size
5 Percent		Cottonseed oil	1 tablespoon
Almond oil	1 tablespoon	Hazelnuts	1/4 cup
Macadamia nuts	1/4 cup	Sunflower seeds	1/4 cup
Safflower oil	1 tablespoon	Wheat germ, toasted	1/4 cup
Soybeans, cooked	1/2 cup	**20 Percent**	
Sweet potato, baked	1 medium	Corn oil	1 tablespoon
10 Percent		Soybean oil	1 tablespoon
Almonds	1/4 cup	**50 Percent**	
Canola oil	1 tablespoon	Wheat-germ oil	1 tablespoon

What circumstances might affect the amount of vitamin E you need to take in each day?

Some lifestyle or health factors can affect the amount of vitamin E you consume or decrease the amount that your body is able to absorb and use. You'll have to be particularly conscientious about taking in the ODA of vitamin E if:

- You have a condition that interferes with fat absorption, such as cystic fibrosis, pancreatitis, biliary cirrhosis, or Crohn's disease.

- You take certain medications, including cholesterol-lowering drugs and mineral oil.

- You smoke cigarettes.

- You are exposed to environmental pollution.

- You have a high intake of PUFAs.

- You are on a low-fat, low-calorie diet to lose weight.

- You are pregnant or breast-feeding.

Is it possible to consume the optimal amount of vitamin E through diet alone?

Almost everyone will need to take vitamin E supplements to reach the recommended ODA range, since it's almost impossible to take in an optimal dose of this nutrient through dietary sources alone.

Chapter 8

Vitamin K

Vitamin K is quite likely the least known of all the vitamins. In fact, many people may not have even heard of this nutrient. Yet, this important vitamin plays a key role in some of the body's most vital functions, including blood clotting.

As with the other vitamins that we have discussed so far, vitamin K is not a single nutrient; it actually exists in three different forms. Two of these forms occur naturally. One natural compound is called K_1—also known as *phylloquinone*—and is found in foods. The other, known as K_2—also called *menaquinone*—is manufactured by bacteria that inhabit the intestinal tract. There is also a synthetic form known as K_3—or *menadione*—that is a more active form of vitamin K.

FUNCTIONS IN THE BODY

Vitamin K is an essential component in the synthesis of proteins involved in the coagulation, or clotting, of blood. The liver uses vitamin K to manufacture prothrombin, which is an important blood-clotting factor.

There is also evidence that vitamin K is necessary for proper bone formation. It helps the protein osteocalcin crystallize calcium in the bones, thereby promoting hardening of the bones.

DEFICIENCY SYMPTOMS

Vitamin K deficiencies are rare, largely because the vitamin is

The History of Vitamin K

Much of our knowledge concerning vitamin K dates back to studies conducted in Denmark in the late 1920s and 1930s. Dr. Hendrik Dam found that chickens fed restricted diets bled spontaneously, and their blood was slow to clot—if it clotted at all. The doctor guessed that the condition was related to a deficiency of a fat-soluble vitamin, and the problem was rectified when the chickens received a particular fat-soluble nutrient. By 1940, Dr. Dam had isolated the nutrient and called it vitamin K for *Koagulationsvitamin,* the Danish spelling for the vitamin that causes blood clotting.

found in a wide variety of foods, and also because it can be manufactured naturally by intestinal bacteria. However, some people are prone to deficits. Vitamin K levels in the body may drop because of the use of antibiotics, which can destroy the vitamin-manufacturing bacteria in the intestines.

Adults and older children can compensate for low levels of vitamin K by adding more K-rich foods to their diets, or by supplementing with the nutrient. However, newborns have an increased risk of deficiency because intestinal bacteria are not present in sufficient numbers to make the vitamin. Plus, infants who are breast-fed receive relatively small amounts of the vitamin from their mothers, because breast milk is not a good source of vitamin K. These days, hospitals routinely administer vitamin K injections, before infants are taken home, to prevent deficiencies.

Symptoms of vitamin K deficiency include abnormal blood clotting and an increased tendency to bleed. Individuals who are deficient in this vitamin may experience nosebleeds, as well as bleeding in the gastrointestinal and urinary tracts.

TOXICITY SYMPTOMS

Vitamins K_1 and K_2—the naturally occurring forms of vitamin K—rarely cause toxic symptoms. However, the synthetic K_3 form *is* potentially toxic. When consumed in excessive amounts, this form of vitamin K has been associated with *hemolytic anemia,* in which red blood cells die more quickly than the body can replace them. The vitamin can also cause impaired liver function in people who already have advanced liver disease.

An excess of K_3 has been linked to jaundice in infants. Jaundice is a yellow discoloration of the skin caused by the buildup of bilirubin, a byproduct of the normal breakdown of red blood cells. Jaundice can lead to deafness and severe neurological problems such as mental retardation.

OPTIMAL DAILY ALLOWANCE

The Optimal Daily Allowance of vitamin K for men and women is 120 micrograms. This amount is higher than the current RDA, which is 60 micrograms daily for women and 80 micrograms daily for men over twenty-five.

Food Sources

About half of the body's requirement of vitamin K is manufactured by bacteria that are present in the intestinal tract. The rest should be consumed from dietary sources. Spinach, turnip greens, broccoli, green cabbage, tomatoes, and liver are some of the best food sources of vitamin K. Significant amounts are also found in meat, milk and other dairy products, eggs, breakfast cereals, and fruits.

Vitamin K is not soluble in water and is quite resistant to heat during cooking; however, it can be destroyed by exposure to light.

Are You Maximizing Your Vitamin K Intake?

Because vitamin K is present in many common foods, most people already take in adequate amounts of the nutrient through their diet. One study concluded that healthy adults consume an average of 300 to 500 micrograms of dietary vitamin K daily—well above the RDA and the ODA of this nutrient. Where do you stand?

You can use the information in Table 8.1 to determine your average daily intake of vitamin K. The foods and beverages included in this table are arranged according to the percentage of the Optimal Daily Allowance of vitamin K they contain. Start by keeping a food diary for at least three to four days; the longer you keep

---

Are You at Risk of Vitamin K Deficiency?

How do you know if you're at risk of vitamin K deficiency? Take a moment to review the questions below. If you answer yes to any of these questions, you have an above-average risk of developing a deficiency.

❏ *Do you have one of the following chronic disorders: liver disease, ulcerative colitis, sprue, or Crohn's disease?* These conditions interfere with the absorption of vitamin K from the intestines and the storage of the vitamin in the body.

❏ *Do you take cholesterol-lowering medications?* Cholesterol-lowering agents—including cholestyramine and colestipol—can diminish the body's ability to absorb vitamin K.

❏ *Do you use mineral oil as a laxative?* The use of mineral oil may cause a vitamin K deficiency because fat-soluble vitamins dissolve in the indigestible oil and are excreted.

❏ *Are you currently taking antibiotics?* Certain antibiotics, including tetracycline, neomycin, and cephalosporin, suppress bacterial production of vitamin K.

---

the diary, the more accurate your calculations will be. Write down everything you eat and drink, as well as the estimated serving size, and refer to the table on page 97 to determine the percentage of the ODA that each food or beverage provides. At the end of the day, add up all of the percentages to see if you've reached 100 percent for the day.

If you find that, on average, you do not take in 100 percent of your ODA for vitamin K, then you may decide that you want to take vitamin supplements for optimal health. But how much of these nutrients do you need to take to reach the ODA? Here's an example of how to perform this calculation: Let's say you discover that you're getting 50 percent (0.50) of your intake target through diet alone. Multiply 0.50 and 120 micrograms (the ODA of vitamin K), and you'll find that you're consuming 60 micrograms of vitamin K in your diet. To make up the difference, then, you should take in 60 micrograms of vitamin K in supplement form.

Table 8.1. Percent of Vitamin K ODA in Common Foods and Beverages

Food	Serving Size	Food	Serving Size
5 Percent		**50 Percent**	
Corn, yellow	$1/2$ cup	Chicken liver	3 ounces
Orange	1 medium	**60 Percent**	
Watercress	$1/2$ cup	Pork liver	3 ounces
10 Percent		**70 Percent**	
Green beans	$1/2$ cup	Beef liver	3 ounces
15 Percent		Coffee	1 cup
Carrots	1 cup	Peas, green, boiled	$3 1/2$ ounces
Strawberries	1 cup	**90 Percent**	
Tomato	$1/2$ cup	Broccoli	1 cup
20 Percent		**100 Percent or More**	
Egg	1 large	Garbanzo beans	$3 1/2$ ounces
Oats	$1/2$ cup	Green tea	1 cup
Soybean oil	1 teaspoon	Lentils	$3 1/2$ ounces
40 Percent		Soybeans	$3 1/2$ ounces
Asparagus	1 cup	Turnip greens	$1/2$ cup
Green cabbage	$1/2$ cup		

Be aware that you might have trouble finding single-dose vita-min K supplements that contain the precise dosage you need to achieve the ODA. Some health food stores sell vitamin K in 100-microgram capsules, but single-dose supplements are not readily available in every community. If you can't find vitamin K supple-ments, look for a quality multivitamin that contains the approxi-mate amount of vitamin K appropriate for your needs.

RECOMMENDATIONS

When it comes to nutrition, there's a lot of important information to remember—so it helps to have what you need to know right at your fingertips. The most critical facts about vitamin K are sum-marized below.

What is the Optimal Daily Allowance of vitamin K?
The ODA of vitamin K for men and women is 120 micrograms.

What circumstances might affect the amount of vitamin K you need to take in each day?
Some lifestyle or health factors can affect the amount of vitamin K you consume or decrease the amount that your body is able to absorb and use. You'll have to be particularly conscientious about taking in the ODA of vitamin K if you have a condition that interferes with the absorption of vitamin K, such as liver disease, ulcerative colitis, sprue, or Crohn's disease. Additionally, the use of some medications, including cholesterol-lowering drugs, mineral oil, and antibiotics, will affect the levels of vitamin K in your body.

Is it possible to consume the optimal amount of vitamin K through diet alone?
According to the U.S. Department of Agriculture and other sources, it is possible to take in enough vitamin K to promote optimal health from dietary sources. In fact, because the vitamin is found in many common foods, most people already take in amounts exceeding the ODA.

Chapter 9

Vitamin B$_1$ (Thiamin)

Vitamin B$_1$, also known as thiamin, was isolated in the mid-1920s, and it has the distinction of being the first B vitamin to be discovered. Along with the other vitamins in the B-complex family, thiamin facilitates the work of every cell in the body.

FUNCTIONS IN THE BODY

Today we know that vitamin B$_1$ is necessary for carbohydrate metabolism. It also helps maintain healthy nervous system function, and there is evidence that it's involved in the production of chemical messengers in the brain known as neurotransmitters.

DEFICIENCY SYMPTOMS

Severe thiamin deficiency can result in the development of *beriberi*, a disease that causes a number of diverse symptoms. Beriberi's effects on the nervous system can include loss of muscle strength, leg spasms, and leg muscle paralysis. Psychological disturbances, such as mental confusion and depression, may also be brought about by this deficiency disease.

Beriberi was first observed in the Far East, where rice is a staple of the diet. Prior to the advent of the milling process in the nineteenth century, unpolished rice was the principal dietary source of thiamin. When milling became common, however, the thiamin-deficiency disease became rampant among Asian populations that consumed the highly polished, refined rice from which

Are You at Risk of Thiamin Deficiency?

How do you know if you're at risk of thiamin deficiency? Take a moment to review the questions below. If you answer yes to any of these questions, you have an above-average risk of developing a deficiency.

❏ *Do you have diabetes?* One symptom of diabetes is *polyuria,* or excessive urination. Because water-soluble vitamins are excreted out of the body in the urine, excessive urination can cause the excessive loss of vitamins such as thiamin.

❏ *Do you have a disorder that increases your metabolic rate?* Hyperthyroidism is known to increase metabolism and, in the short term, fever has the same effect. Thiamin requirements are greater during periods of increased metabolism.

❏ *Do you consume large amounts of alcohol?* Alcohol reduces the absorption of thiamin in the intestines. Also, alcoholics tend to substitute alcohol—which has no real nutritional value—for nutrient-dense foods, so they generally don't take in adequate amounts of thiamin and other nutrients.

❏ *Is your diet high in carbohydrates?* Thiamin is necessary for carbohydrate metabolism for energy. Therefore, the more carbohydrates you consume, the more thiamin your body needs to use the carbohydrates effectively.

❏ *Do you regularly include raw fish in your diet?* Thiamin is inactivated by an enzyme called thiaminase that is found in raw fish. The enzyme is destroyed by heat, however, so cooking fish eliminates this problem.

❏ *Are you pregnant or breast-feeding?* Pregnancy is a time of increased nutritional needs because the growth of a new person requires every known nutrient. The National Research Council recommends that pregnant women take in an additional 0.4 milligrams of vitamin B_1 daily. Women who are breast-feeding should increase their intake by 0.5 milligrams daily to compensate for the amount that is contained in breast milk. The ODA of vitamin B_1 is more than adequate to meet the increased needs of women who are pregnant or breast-feeding.

the vitamin-rich husks had been removed. As with so many other diseases brought on by vitamin deficiencies, investigators at first tried to identify a microbial cause of the disease. It wasn't until the turn of the century that rice bran, in which vitamin B_1 is contained, was found to alleviate the symptoms of beriberi.

People who live in developed countries are relatively safe from vitamin B_1 deficiency and beriberi, due to the wide availability of a variety of foods that contain the vitamin. Individuals who abuse alcohol are most likely to develop deficiency symptoms for two reasons. First, the more alcohol a person drinks, the less likely it is that he or she will eat enough food to obtain adequate nutrients. Second, alcohol interferes with the body's absorption of thiamin.

TOXICITY SYMPTOMS

There are no known symptoms of toxicity associated with high doses of thiamin when the nutrient is taken orally. However, high doses administered intravenously have produced severe allergic reactions, including anaphylactic shock.

OPTIMAL DAILY ALLOWANCE

The ODA of thiamin ranges from 1.5 to 10 milligrams. The lowest recommended intake is acceptable for many people, but the higher end of the range is more appropriate for individuals who are extremely active, and for people who consume high-carbohydrate diets. Higher levels of thiamin consumption are also important for men and women who have liver disease or who are at increased risk for liver disease because of excessive alcohol consumption. Individuals who are at risk of deficiency due to conditions such as diabetes or hyperthyroidism must be especially careful to take in at least 1.5 milligrams daily.

Food Sources

Vitamin B_1 is present in many foods. Some of the best sources of the vitamin include whole-grain or enriched breads and cereals, brewer's yeast, liver and other organ meats, lean cuts of pork, peas, beans, and nuts and seeds.

Exposure to light can destroy some of the thiamin content of foods. Heat can also cause foods to lose a portion of the nutrient, so baking, broiling, or roasting can reduce the amount of the vitamin in foods. Boiling seems to deplete vitamin B_1 levels more than any other method of food preparation, because the cooking water actually leeches some of the nutrient from foods. To retain most of the original content of this water-soluble vitamin, cook vitamin B_1-containing foods in small amounts of water.

Are You Maximizing Your Thiamin Intake?

Statistics have shown that many people in the United States do reach the lower end of the ODA range for vitamin B_1 through dietary sources alone, and many others come close to this intake. Surveys taken in 1994 found that men consume an average of 1.93 milligrams of thiamin per day, while women average an intake of 1.31 milligrams. However, for all of the individuals who take in 1.5 milligrams or more daily, there are many others who do not reach even the minimum ODA, and who would benefit from supplementation. Where do you stand?

You can use the information in Table 9.1 to determine your average daily intake of vitamin B_1. The foods and beverages included in this table are arranged according to the percentage of the Optimal Daily Allowance of vitamin B_1 they contain. Remember, the ODA of vitamin B_1 ranges from 1.5 to 10 milligrams. For this self-test, we'll use the lowest ODA in the range, 1.5 milligrams.

Start by keeping a food diary for at least three to four days; the longer you keep the diary, the more accurate your calculations will be. Write down everything you eat and drink, as well as the estimated serving size, and refer to the table on page 104 to determine the percentage of the ODA that each food or beverage provides. At the end of the day, add up all of the percentages to see if you've reached 100 percent for the day. (If your optimal dose falls elsewhere in our recommended range, take that into account when calculating percentages.)

If you find that, on average, you do not take in 100 percent of your ODA for vitamin B_1, then you may decide that you want to take vitamin supplements for optimal health. But how much of this nutrient do you need to take to reach your ODA? Here's an

Table 9.1. Percent of Thiamin ODA in Common Foods and Beverages

Food	Serving Size	Food	Serving Size
5 Percent		Garbanzo beans, boiled	1 cup
Avocado, California	1/2 medium	Great Northern beans,	
Bacon, cooked	3 slices	boiled	1 cup
Beef		Kidney beans, boiled	1 cup
flank steak, broiled	3 1/2 ounces	Mackerel	3 ounces
top round, broiled	3 1/2 ounces	Orange juice	
Bread, white or wheat	1 slice	from concentrate	8 ounces
Figs, dried	10 figs	Peanuts	1 ounce
Grapefruit juice, canned	1 cup	Peas, green, boiled	1/2 cup
Hazelnuts	1 ounce	Pecans	1 ounce
Lamb, leg of, roasted	3 ounces	Pistachio nuts	1 ounce
Macadamia nuts	1 ounce	Potato, baked	
Mango	1 medium	without skin	1 medium
Marinara sauce	1 cup	Rice, brown or white	
Milk, 1%	1 cup	(enriched), cooked	1 cup
Miso	1/2 cup	Salmon	3 ounces
Orange	1 medium	Spaghetti (enriched),	
Pineapple juice,		cooked	1 cup
canned	1 cup	Tortilla, corn	1 tortilla
Tofu	1/2 cup	**20 Percent**	
Yogurt, low-fat	8 ounces	Black beans, boiled	1 cup
10 Percent		Black-eyed peas, boiled	1 cup
Acorn squash, baked	1/2 cup	Bran Flakes cereal	1 ounce
Avocado, Florida	1/2 medium	Corn Flakes cereal	1 ounce
Bagel	1 bagel	Cream of Wheat,	
Beef liver, braised	3 1/2 ounces	instant	1 packet
Brazil nuts	1 ounce	Lentils, boiled	1 cup
Broad beans, boiled	1 cup	Lima beans, boiled	1 cup
Carrot juice, canned	6 ounce	Navy beans, boiled	1 cup
Chicken liver, simmered	3 1/2 ounces	Pinto beans, boiled	1 cup
Corn, yellow, boiled	1/2 cup	Raisin Bran cereal	1 ounce
		Trout	3 ounces

Food	Serving Size	Food	Serving Size
30 Percent		Sunflower seeds	1 ounce
Oatmeal, instant	1 packet	**60 Percent**	
Pork shoulder, roasted	3½ ounces	Ham, canned	3½ ounces
Wheat germ, toasted	½ cup	**100 Percent or More**	
40 Percent		Brewer's yeast	1 ounce
Baker's yeast, dry	1 ounce	Product 19 cereal	1 ounce
Pork loin, roasted	3½ ounces	Total cereal	1 ounce

example of how to perform this calculation: Let's say you determine that you are getting 60 percent (0.60) of your target intake through diet alone. Multiply 0.60 and 1.5 milligrams (the ODA of thiamin) and you'll find that you're consuming 0.9 milligrams of thiamin in your diet. To make up the difference, then, you should take in 0.6 milligrams of thiamin in supplement form.

Most multivitamins contain at least the low end of the ODA of thiamin, and often more—so if you take a multivitamin tablet each day, you're probably getting all the extra thiamin you need. This vitamin is nontoxic, even in large doses, so you won't be putting yourself at any risk, even if you take more than the ODA.

RECOMMENDATIONS

When it comes to nutrition, there's a lot of important information to remember—so it helps to have what you need to know right at your fingertips. The most critical facts about thiamin are summarized below.

What is the Optimal Daily Allowance of thiamin?
The ODA of thiamin for men and women ranges from 1.5 to 10 milligrams.

What circumstances might affect the amount of thiamin you need to take in each day?
Some lifestyle or health factors can affect the amount of thiamin you consume or decrease the amount that your body is able to

absorb and use. You'll have to be particularly conscientious about taking in the ODA of thiamin if:

- You have diabetes.

- You have a metabolic disorder, such as hyperthyroidism.

- You eat a high-carbohydrate diet.

- You include a lot of raw fish in your diet.

- You drink large amounts of alcohol.

- You are pregnant or breast-feeding.

Is it possible to consume the optimal amount of thiamin through diet alone?

It's certainly possible to reach the lower end of the ODA range for thiamin through dietary sources alone, and many people in the United States do take in the minimum allowance for this vitamin. In fact, surveys show that the average man consumes more than the minimum ODA, and the average woman comes close. However, these are averages—there are also many people who do not take in these amounts, and who would therefore benefit from supplementation. Furthermore, people who are aiming for the higher end of the ODA range—because of lifestyle factors or health conditions that increase their risk of deficiency—will find that it's almost impossible to take in these amounts through diet alone.

Chapter 10

Vitamin B$_2$ (Riboflavin)

Vitamin B$_2$ was first identified when researchers noted a yellow fluorescent concentrate in milk whey. Within a short time, the yellow pigment was also discovered in other food sources, including liver and eggs. When the nutrient was finally isolated and identified in the 1930s, researchers called it *riboflavin*, which takes its root from the Latin word *flavius*, meaning yellow.

FUNCTIONS IN THE BODY

Like the other B vitamins, riboflavin is important for energy production in the body. It is part of two coenzymes involved in the metabolism of carbohydrates, fats, and proteins. This vitamin is also essential for the normal growth and repair of all body tissues.

DEFICIENCY SYMPTOMS

Studies have shown that taking in less than 0.55 milligrams daily of riboflavin can cause a deficiency. Initial signs tend to be general in nature, including loss of appetite and reduced growth. This is followed by the appearance of localized deficiency symptoms, such as sores, cracks, and dry or scaly skin on the nose, lips, and corners of the mouth; inflamed tongue and loss of the sense of taste; eye disorders, such as tearing, burning, reddened eyes and a decrease in the sharpness of vision; and anemia. Changes in behavior—including depression, nervousness, and irritability—may also result from damage to the nervous system. It's important to note that these symptoms won't develop overnight, because the kidneys and liver store small amounts of B_2. In fact, a deficiency may not become apparent for some three to four months.

Are You at Risk of Riboflavin Deficiency?

How do you know if you're at risk of riboflavin deficiency? Take a moment to review the questions below. If you answer yes to any of these questions, you have an above-average risk of developing a deficiency.

❏ *Do you have diabetes?* One symptom of diabetes is *polyuria,* or excessive urination. Because water-soluble vitamins are excreted out of the body in the urine, excessive urination can cause the excessive loss of vitamins such as riboflavin.

❏ *Do you use diuretics?* Diuretics cause increased water excretion, and with it, increased losses of water-soluble vitamins such as vitamin B_2 in the urine.

❏ *Do you take phobenecid for gout?* Phobenecid causes vitamin B_2 to be excreted in the urine.

❏ *Do you take tricyclic antidepressants?* Tricyclic antidepressant medications can inhibit riboflavin metabolism.

❏ *Do you exercise regularly?* Exercising augments the body's need for vitamin B_2 because the nutrient is an important factor in energy production. Even moderate activity requires increased intake of the vitamin.

❏ *Are you pregnant or breast-feeding?* Pregnancy is a time of increased nutritional needs because the growth of a new person requires every known nutrient. The National Research Council recommends that pregnant women take in an additional 0.3 milligrams of vitamin B_2 daily. Women who are breast-feeding should increase their intake by 0.5 milligrams daily during the first six months, and 0.4 milligrams each day for longer periods of breast-feeding, to compensate for the amount that is contained in breast milk. The ODA of vitamin B_2 is more than adequate to meet the increased needs of women who are pregnant or breast-feeding.

Because riboflavin is necessary for vitamin B_6 and niacin to carry out their functions in the body, a vitamin B_2 deficiency can also produce symptoms related to shortages of these other B vitamins. (See Chapters 11 and 13 for information about the symptoms of these deficiencies.)

TOXICITY SYMPTOMS

Taking excessive amounts of riboflavin has no known adverse effects.

OPTIMAL DAILY ALLOWANCE

The Optimal Daily Allowance of riboflavin for men and women is 2 to 5 milligrams. If you are extremely active, or if you consume large amounts of carbohydrates for energy, you should probably take in amounts from the higher end of the range—4 or 5 milligrams.

Food Sources

Milk and other dairy foods, including cheese, ice cream, and yogurt, are rich sources of vitamin B_2; however, the higher the fat content of a dairy food, the less riboflavin it contains. Meat (especially liver and other organ meats), poultry, and fish (including salmon and tuna) are also high in riboflavin. Other good sources include avocados, broccoli, Brussels sprouts, and spinach. Although cereals and grains naturally contain little B_2, they are often enriched with the vitamin.

Exposure to sunlight can greatly reduce the riboflavin content of foods. Therefore, it's important to store riboflavin-rich foods away from sunlight—in the refrigerator, in cupboards, and/or in opaque containers. Cooking foods can also deplete their levels of vitamin B_2.

Are You Maximizing Your Riboflavin Intake?

The U.S. Department of Agriculture has reported that men take in an average of 2.25 milligrams of vitamin B_2 daily, while women average 1.57 milligrams daily. However, these figures are only averages, which suggests that many people actually fall short of reaching the ODA, and will therefore benefit from supplementation. In addition, people who need to take in amounts from the higher end of the ODA range will find that supplementation with vitamin B$_2$ is absolutely essential.

You can use the information in Table 10.1 to determine your average daily intake of vitamin B$_2$. The foods and beverages included in this table are arranged according to the percentage of the Optimal Daily Allowance of vitamin B$_2$ they contain. Remember, the ODA of riboflavin ranges from 2 to 5 milligrams. For this self-test, we'll use the lowest ODA in the range, 2 milligrams.

Start by keeping a food diary for at least three to four days; the longer you keep the diary, the more accurate your calculations will be. Write down everything you eat and drink, as well as the estimated serving size, and refer to the table on page 111 to determine the percentage of the ODA that each food or beverage provides. At the end of each day, add up all of the percentages to see if you've reached 100 percent for the day. (If your optimal dose falls elsewhere in the recommended range, take that into account when calculating percentages.)

If you find that, on average, you do not take in 100 percent of your ODA for riboflavin, then you may decide that you want to take vitamin supplements for optimal health. But how much of this nutrient do you need to take to reach your ODA? Here's an example of how to perform this calculation: Let's say that you determine that you are getting 60 percent (0.60) of your target intake through diet alone. Multiply 60 percent and 2 milligrams (the ODA of riboflavin) and you'll find that you're consuming 1.2 milligrams of riboflavin in your diet. To make up the difference, then, you should take in 0.8 milligrams of the vitamin in supplement form.

RECOMMENDATIONS

When it comes to nutrition, there's a lot of important information to remember—so it helps to have what you need to know right at your fingertips. The most critical facts about riboflavin are summarized below.

Table 10.1. Percent of Riboflavin ODA in Common Foods and Beverages

Food	Serving Size	Food	Serving Size
5 Percent		Lima beans, boiled	1 cup
American cheese	1 ounce	Limburger cheese	1 ounce
Apple, dried	10 rings	Marinara sauce	1 cup
Asparagus, boiled	6 spears	Monterey Jack cheese	1 ounce
Avocado, California	$\frac{1}{2}$ medium	Mushrooms	$\frac{1}{2}$ cup
Bagel	1 bagel	Navy beans, boiled	1 cup
Beef, brisket, braised	$3\frac{1}{2}$ ounces	Oysters	6 medium
Beef soup, chunky	1 cup	Peas, green, boiled	$\frac{1}{2}$ cup
Black beans, boiled	1 cup	Pinto beans, boiled	1 cup
Blue cheese	1 ounce	Prunes, dried	10 prunes
Brie cheese	1 ounce	Sweet potato, baked	1 medium
Broad beans, boiled	1 cup	Swiss cheese	1 ounce
Broccoli, boiled	$\frac{1}{2}$ cup	Turkey, light meat, roasted	$3\frac{1}{2}$ ounces
Cheddar cheese	1 ounce		
Chicken		**10 Percent**	
breast meat, roasted	$\frac{1}{2}$ breast	Almonds	1 ounce
light meat, roasted	$3\frac{1}{2}$ ounces	Anchovies	3 ounces
thigh meat, roasted	1 thigh		
wing meat, roasted	1 wing	Avocado, Florida	$\frac{1}{2}$ medium
Chicken soup, chunky	1 cup	Beef	
Colby cheese	1 ounce	bottom round, braised	$3\frac{1}{2}$ ounces
Corned beef, cooked	$3\frac{1}{2}$ ounces	flank steak	$3\frac{1}{2}$ ounces
		ground (lean), baked	$3\frac{1}{2}$ ounces
Cream of Wheat, instant	1 packet	top round, braised	$3\frac{1}{2}$ ounces
Egg	1 large	Beet greens	$\frac{1}{2}$ cup
Figs, dried	10 figs	Chicken	
Garbanzo beans, boiled	1 cup	dark meat, roasted	$3\frac{1}{2}$ ounces
Gouda cheese	1 ounce	leg meat, roasted	1 leg
Great Northern beans, boiled	1 cup	Clams	4 large or 9 small
Kidney beans, boiled	1 cup	Ham, canned	$3\frac{1}{2}$ ounces
Lamb		Herring	3 ounces
loin chop, broiled	1 chop	Ice cream, vanilla	1 cup
rib chop, broiled	1 chop	Ice milk, vanilla	1 cup

Food	Serving Size	Food	Serving Size
Lamb, leg of, roasted	3 ounces	Buttermilk	1 cup
Mackerel	3 ounces	Corn Flakes cereal	1 ounce
Miso	1/2 cup	Cottage cheese, low-fat	1 cup
Oatmeal, instant	1 packet	Milk, 1%	1 cup
Peaches, dried	10 halves	Pudding, vanilla	1 cup
Pears, dried	10 halves	Raisin Bran cereal	1 ounce
Pork		Yogurt, low-fat	8 ounces
loin, roasted	3 1/2 ounces	**70 Percent**	
shoulder, roasted	3 1/2 ounces	Brewer's yeast	1 ounce
Prune juice, canned	1 cup	**90 Percent**	
Ricotta cheese, part-skim	4 ounces	Baker's yeast, dry	1 ounce
Salmon	3 ounces	Chicken liver, simmered	3 1/2 ounces
Trout	3 ounces	Product 19 cereal	1 ounce
Turkey, dark meat, roasted	3 1/2 ounces	Total cereal	1 ounce
Wheat germ, toasted	1/4 cup	**100 Percent or More**	
20 Percent		Beef liver, braised	3 1/2 ounces
Bran Flakes cereal	1 ounce		

What is the Optimal Daily Allowance of riboflavin?
The ODA of riboflavin for men and women ranges from 2 to 5 milligrams.

What circumstances might affect the amount of riboflavin you need to take in each day?
Some lifestyle or health factors can affect the amount of riboflavin you consume or decrease the amount that your body is able to absorb and use. You'll have to be particularly conscientious about taking in the ODA of riboflavin if:

• You have diabetes.

• You take certain medications, including diuretics, phobenecid, or tricyclic antidepressants.

• You exercise regularly.

• You're pregnant or breast-feeding.

Is it possible to consume the optimal amount of riboflavin through diet alone?

Surveys show that, on average, men take in at least the minimum ODA of riboflavin from dietary sources, and women tend to come close. However, there are also many people who need a supplement to reach even the minimum allowance. And individuals who are aiming to take in amounts from the higher end of the ODA range—because of lifestyle or health factors—will find that supplementation is virtually essential to achieve these intakes.

Chapter 11

Vitamin B$_3$ (Niacin)

Vitamin B$_3$, also called niacin, was once a relatively obscure nutrient, probably best known in medical circles for its role in preventing *pellagra*, a deficiency disease that affects the skin, the gastrointestinal tract, and the central nervous system. Today, we know that vitamin B$_3$ has other important functions in the body, as well. In the 1980s, the nutrient gained widespread acclaim as a potential weapon in the battle against cardiovascular disease, specifically for its ability to lower blood cholesterol levels.

There are two natural, active forms of niacin: *nicotinic acid* and *nicotinamide* (also called *niacinamide*). While these two compounds may sound similar in name to nicotine, they are not chemically related to the harmful "soundalike." To avoid any confusion that may result, however, the more generic term niacin is often used to represent both nicotinic acid and nicotinamide.

FUNCTIONS IN THE BODY

Niacin functions as a coenzyme in many of the body's vital metabolic processes, including energy production. More specifically, it aids in the metabolism of carbohydrates, fats, and proteins, helping to convert the energy in these macronutrients into a form the body can use. These reactions take place in every cell in the body, and as such, a niacin deficiency—or any B vitamin deficiency, for that matter—affects all of the body's cells.

In large doses, the nicotinic acid form of vitamin B$_3$ decreases total blood levels of cholesterol, as well as levels of "bad" low-density lipoprotein (LDL) cholesterol. It also can reduce blood levels of triglycerides. The nutrient has been shown to increase blood levels of "good" high-density lipoprotein (HDL) cholesterol, as well.

HEALTH BENEFITS

Back in the 1980s, vitamin B_3 was recognized for its role in helping to lower total blood cholesterol levels. In fact, the evidence for this benefit was so persuasive that the government's Expert Panel of the National Cholesterol Education Program listed nicotinic acid among the primary drugs that doctors should recommend first to control cholesterol levels. The members of the Panel were particularly impressed by studies that indicated a significant drop in the risk of heart disease corresponding to reduced cholesterol levels.

One of the best known clinical trials of niacin's effects on cholesterol dates back to the 1970s. The Coronary Drug Project, as the study was called, involved approximately 5,000 men with a history of coronary heart disease who were randomly assigned to receive one of three treatments. One group of men took 3 grams of niacin daily to control their cholesterol levels; a second group took a cholesterol-lowering medication called clofibrate; and the rest of the men took a placebo, with no active ingredients. The results of the study showed that after five years, the participants taking niacin had the lowest average cholesterol levels—226 milligrams per deciliter (mg/dl). Those men taking clofibrate had average measurements of 235 mg/dl, while 251 was the average measurement for men in the placebo group. Equally impressive was the finding that men taking niacin had fewer life-threatening coronary events such as heart attacks. The percentage of men from the niacin group who experienced coronary events was 19.8 percent lower than in the placebo group. Among the participants taking clofibrate, there was only a 9.5 percent reduction in the incidence of coronary events, when compared with the placebo group.

Note: Nicotinic acid functions as a drug, rather than as a vitamin, when taken in the high doses necessary to reduce cholesterol levels. As such, it should be taken at these levels only under the advice and supervision of a health-care professional. Your doctor can order periodic blood tests to be sure that the high doses of

The History of Niacin

The history of niacin extends back to the early 1900s, and begins with research conducted on a debilitating disease known as pellagra. Pellagra had been recognized as far back as the eighteenth century, but its cause remained unidentified. The disease has three characteristic symptoms: dermatitis, diarrhea, and dementia. Left untreated, it can cause death.

Pellagra is relatively rare today, but it affected approximately two hundred thousand Americans each year in the early twentieth century. At that time, many scientists were convinced that an infectious agent was responsible for the disease and, in their research, they sought to identify a disease-causing microbe. As it turned out, this was not the correct approach, and so their attempts did not yield positive results.

Ultimately, a government investigator named Joseph Goldberger began to explore the possibility that a nutritional deficiency was to blame. He set up a study in Jackson, Mississippi, at an orphanage with a high incidence of pellagra among the children. Goldberger found that the children's symptoms disappeared when they were fed high-protein foods like meat, beans, and eggs. At first, he concluded that a protein deficiency caused pellagra. Finally, in the 1930s, researchers identified a vitamin, niacin, as the factor in the high-protein foods that reversed the symptoms of pellagra.

Ironically, some of the high-protein foods that Goldberger gave the children in his study contain little niacin. Rather, those foods are rich in the amino acid *tryptophan,* which is converted to niacin in the body. Now we know that the body's ability to convert tryptophan to niacin helps us meet our daily requirement.

niacin are not adversely affecting your liver function. These visits to your doctor's office are extremely important and are well worth the time and expense.

DEFICIENCY SYMPTOMS

The symptoms seen most frequently among individuals who are

Are You at Risk of Niacin Deficiency?

How do you know if you're at risk of niacin deficiency? Take a moment to review the questions below. If you answer yes to any of these questions, you have an above-average risk of developing a deficiency.

❏ *Do you exercise regularly?* The more energy you expend, the more niacin you need, because niacin plays a role in converting foods into energy.

❏ *Are you pregnant or breast-feeding?* Pregnancy is a time of increased nutritional needs because the growth of a new person requires every known nutrient. The National Research Council recommends that pregnant women take in an additional 2 milligrams of vitamin B_3 daily. Women who are breast-feeding also need extra vitamin B_3 to compensate for the amount that is contained in breast milk, and because they expend more energy in the form of calories. The ODA of vitamin B_3 is more than adequate to meet the increased needs of women who are pregnant or breast-feeding.

vitamin B_3 deficient are skin disorders. The skin becomes dry, cracked, and scaly, and may appear to be darkly pigmented, particularly in areas exposed to sunlight, including the forehead, neck, and backs of the hands. Niacin deficiency also affects the nervous system, leading to irritability, anxiety, depression, tremors, muscle weakness, confusion, and disorientation. In the most severe cases, dementia and hallucinations may result.

The deficiency disease pellagra is rare these days, but it does affect some populations living in parts of the world where both niacin- and tryptophan-rich foods are scarce and where diets are poor. Symptoms of severe deficiency and pellagra include dermatitis (an inflammation of the skin that produces scaling, flaking, and color changes), diarrhea, delirium, and swelling of the mouth and tongue. If the deficiency is not remedied, pellagra can result in death.

TOXICITY SYMPTOMS

Overall, the risk of vitamin B_3 toxicity is low if you stick with the doses contained in most vitamin supplements. Intake of the nicotinic acid form of vitamin B_3 may cause what is known as "niacin flush," a condition that makes the skin turn red, usually within an hour or two after the supplement is taken. This occurs because the nicotinic acid stimulates the release of histamine, a substance that causes the blood vessels to dilate. According to one study, 92 percent of people who take doses of 3 grams per day experience this flushing. While this makes some individuals uncomfortable enough to discontinue use of the vitamin, many other people develop a tolerance to the effect, or are able to control the reaction by taking aspirin or an antihistamine shortly before taking nicotinic acid.

Other side effects associated with a high nicotinic-acid intake include skin tingling, itching, stinging, rashes, headaches, dry skin, nausea, and diarrhea. While these effects are not comfortable, they are generally harmless and reversible. However, in the past, some people who used niacin to reduce blood cholesterol levels developed toxic symptoms because they self-prescribed excessively large amounts of the nutrient. Physicians are much more worried about serious consequences of taking extremely high doses—3 grams a day or more—including high blood sugar levels, ulcers, liver damage, or irregular heart rhythms. A 3-gram (3,000-milligram) dose of nicotinic acid can double a person's risk of developing certain kinds of abnormal heart rhythms and is generally considered to be toxic. Although you can purchase nicotinic acid in supermarkets and pharmacies without a prescription, you should take the potential risks of this substance seriously. Most doctors advise people who have peptic ulcers, diabetes, or liver disease to be particularly cautious when using nicotinic acid.

Fewer serious toxic risks have been associated with nicotinamide than with nicotinic acid, but problems can occur with either form of vitamin B_3. Heartburn, nausea, headaches, fatigue, sore throat, and dry hair have been reported in association with high doses of nicotinamide.

OPTIMAL DAILY ALLOWANCE

The Optimal Daily Allowance of niacin for men and women is 20 milligrams. This amount will meet the needs of even the most active men and women.

As you first read on page 117, the amino acid tryptophan can be converted to niacin in the body, and this process may be adequate to prevent deficiency in many individuals. However, the conversion process may not provide an optimal amount of niacin, so most people need to take in extra amounts of the nutrient to meet the ODA.

Food Sources

Good sources of vitamin B_3 include poultry, fish, and whole-grain and enriched breads. Nuts and legumes are rich in this vitamin as well, as are potatoes and tomatoes. Also, many cereals are enriched with vitamin B_3.

Food sources of the amino acid tryptophan can help meet the body's requirement for vitamin B_3. For example, although milk and eggs have a limited vitamin B_3 content, they are rich in tryptophan. As such, these foods are wise choices for maintaining an optimal intake.

Vitamin B_3 is a stable vitamin that can withstand high temperatures and exposure to oxygen. The nutrient dissolves in water, however, so some of the niacin content of foods may be lost in cooking water. Therefore, it's best to steam, bake, or stir-fry your foods if you wish to retain their vitamin B_3 content.

Are You Maximizing Your Niacin Intake?

Since niacin is available in a variety of common foods, many adult Americans do come close to reaching the ODA of 20 milligrams through dietary sources alone, and some people even exceed this allowance. For example, the government's Continuing Survey of Food Intakes by Individuals for 1994 found that adults consume an average of 22.3 milligrams of this vitamin daily. Other studies have shown that the typical American diet includes 700 milligrams of tryptophan daily for women and 1,100 milligrams daily for men, which provides 11.7 milligrams and 18.4 milligrams of vitamin B_3, respectively. However, these figures only represent average intakes, so for all of the people who take in more than the ODA, there are many others who fall short of this intake. Where do you stand?

You can use the information in Table 11.1 to determine your average daily intake of vitamin B_3. The foods and beverages included in this table are arranged according to the percentage of the Optimal Daily Allowance of vitamin B_3 they contain. Start by keeping a food diary for at least three to four days; the longer you keep the diary, the more accurate your calculations will be. Write down everything you eat and drink, as well as the estimated serving size, and refer to the table on page 122 to determine the percentage of the ODA that each food or drink provides. At the end of the day, add up all of the percentages to see if you've reached 100 percent for the day.

If you find that, on average, you do not take in 100 percent of your ODA for vitamin B_3, then you may decide that you want to take vitamin supplements for optimal health. But how much of this nutrient do you need to take to reach your ODA? Here's an example of how to perform this calculation: Let's say you determine that you are getting 50 percent (0.50) of your target intake through diet alone. Multiply 0.50 and 20 milligrams (the ODA of niacin), and you'll find that you're consuming 10 milligrams of niacin in your diet. To make up the difference, then, you should take in 10 milligrams of niacin in supplement form.

RECOMMENDATIONS

When it comes to nutrition, there's a lot of important information to remember—so it helps to have what you need to know right at your fingertips. The most critical facts about niacin are summarized below.

What is the Optimal Daily Allowance of niacin?
The ODA of niacin for men and women is 20 milligrams.

What circumstances might affect the amount of niacin you need to take in each day?
Some lifestyle factors can affect the amount of niacin you consume or decrease the amount that your body is able to absorb and use. You'll have to be particularly conscientious about taking in the ODA of niacin if you exercise regularly, or if you are pregnant or breast-feeding.

Table 11.1. Percent of Niacin ODA in Common Foods and Beverages

Food	Serving Size	Food	Serving Size
5 Percent		Potato chips	1 ounce
Almonds	1 ounce	Pretzels	1 ounce
Apricots, dried	10 halves	Prunes, dried	10 prunes
Avocado, California	$1/2$ medium	Raisins, golden, seedless	$2/3$ cup
Bacon, cooked	3 slices	Sardines, canned in oil	2 sardines
Bagel	1 bagel	Scallops	6 large/ 14 small
Bread, white or whole wheat	1 slice	Sole	$31/2$ ounces
Broad beans, boiled	1 cup	Spaghetti (enriched), cooked	1 cup
Clams	4 large or 9 small	Sunflower seeds	1 ounce
Cod	3 ounces	Tomato juice, canned	6 ounces
Corn, yellow, boiled	$1/2$ cup	Tortilla, corn	1 tortilla
Crab	3 ounces	Turkey breast	1 slice
Dates, dried	10 dates	Vegetable soup, chunky	1 cup
Figs, dried	10 figs	Wheat germ, toasted	2 ounces
Flounder	$31/2$ ounces	**10 Percent**	
Frankfurter, beef	1 frank	Avocado, Florida	$1/2$ medium
French bread	1 slice	Beef bottom round, braised brisket, braised	$31/2$ ounces $31/2$ ounces
Great Northern beans, boiled	1 cup	Beef soup, chunky	1 cup
Guava	1 medium	Chicken thigh meat, roasted wing meat, roasted	1 thigh 1 wing
Kidney beans, boiled	1 cup	Corned beef	$31/2$ ounces
Lobster	3 ounces	Haddock	3 ounces
Mango	1 medium	Ham, canned	$31/2$ ounces
Manhattan clam chowder	1 cup	Herring	3 ounces
Miso	$1/2$ cup	Lamb, loin chop, broiled	1 chop
Mushrooms	$1/2$ cup	Lentils, boiled	1 cup
Navy beans, boiled	1 cup	Peanut butter	1 tablespoon
Nectarine	1 medium		
Oysters	6 medium		
Peas, green, boiled	$1/2$ cup		

Food	Serving Size	Food	Serving Size
Peanuts	1 ounce	Raisin Bran cereal	1 ounce
Pears, dried	10 halves	Tuna, canned in water	3 ounces
Potato, baked, with or without skin	1 medium	Turkey, light and dark meat, roasted	3¹/₂ ounces
Prune juice, canned	1 cup	**30 Percent**	
Rice, brown or white (enriched), cooked	1 cup	Chicken dark meat, roasted	3¹/₂ ounces
Shrimp	12 large	leg meat, roasted	1 leg
Turkey, dark meat, roasted	3¹/₂ ounces	Mackerel	3 ounces
20 Percent		Salmon	3 ounces
Beef		Turkey, light meat, roasted	3¹/₂ ounces
flank steak	3¹/₂ ounces	**40 Percent**	
ground (lean), baked	3¹/₂ ounces	Chicken, light and dark meat, roasted	3¹/₂ ounces
top round, broiled	3¹/₂ ounces	Swordfish	3 ounces
Bran Flakes cereal	1 ounce	**50 Percent**	
Chicken liver, simmered	3¹/₂ ounces	Anchovies	3 ounces
Chicken soup, chunky	1 cup	Beef liver, braised	3¹/₂ ounces
Corn Flakes cereal	1 ounce	Chicken, light meat, roasted	3¹/₂ ounces
Cream of Wheat, instant	1 packet	**60 Percent**	
Ground beef, baked	3¹/₂ ounces	Chicken, breast meat, roasted	¹/₂ breast
Halibut	3 ounces	**100 Percent or More**	
Lamb, leg of, roasted	3 ounces	Product 19 cereal	1 ounce
Marinara sauce	1 cup	Total cereal	1 ounce
Oatmeal, instant	1 packet		
Peaches, dried	10 halves		
Pork shoulder, roasted	3¹/₂ ounces		

Is it possible to consume the optimal amount of niacin through diet alone? It's possible to consume the ODA of niacin through diet, since this vitamin is found in many common foods. Some surveys have shown that many adults actually exceed their optimal allowance, or at least come close to reaching this intake level. However, for all of those people who take in more than the ODA, there are those who fall short, and may need to supplement with the vitamin.

Chapter 12

Vitamin B$_5$ (Pantothenic Acid)

Pantothenic acid gets its name from the Greek word *pantos*, which means "everywhere." And what an appropriate description! Vitamin B$_5$—as pantothenic acid is sometimes called—is widely available in plant and animal foods. Indeed, at least small amounts of pantothenic acid are present in almost all of the foods we eat.

FUNCTIONS IN THE BODY

Soon after pantothenic acid is consumed, the body converts most of the nutrient to *coenzyme A*, a substance that is required to produce energy from carbohydrates, fats, and some proteins. This B vitamin is also necessary for the body's production of *hormones*, chemicals secreted by the endocrine glands that act as messengers in the body; *hemoglobin*, the oxygen-carrying compound in red blood cells; and the neurotransmitter *acetylcholine*, which transmits nerve impulses from one nerve cell to another. The adrenal glands also depend upon pantothenic acid for proper functioning, so adequate intake is especially important during times of prolonged stress.

HEALTH BENEFITS

Pantothenic acid has no proven uses for treating disease. Some people have claimed that this B vitamin can improve the symptoms caused by rheumatoid arthritis, an autoimmune disorder in which the body's immune system attacks the joints, damaging the cartilage and tissues in and around the joints. However, the limited amount of research that has focused on the use of pantothenic acid for rheumatoid arthritis has not provided support for this claim.

DEFICIENCY SYMPTOMS

All foods contain at least some pantothenic acid, and since the body needs only limited amounts of this nutrient, the risk of a deficiency is minimal. In general, people who are deficient in vitamin B_5 are deficient in all of the other B vitamins, as well.

Because pantothenic acid deficiency is so rare, diseases associated with inadequate intake of this nutrient have not been clearly identified—with one exception. During the 1940s, prisoners of war in the Far East developed severe pain, numbness, and tingling in their feet and toes. The condition was appropriately labeled "burn-

---

Are You at Risk of Vitamin B_5 Deficiency?

How do you know if you're at risk of vitamin B_5 deficiency? Take a moment to review the questions below. If you answer yes to any of these questions, you have an above-average risk of developing a deficiency.

❏ *Do you have diabetes?* One symptom of diabetes is *polyuria,* or excessive urination. Because water-soluble vitamins are excreted out of the body in the urine, excessive urination can cause the excessive loss of vitamins such as pantothenic acid.

❏ *Do you drink large amounts of alcohol?* Alcohol reduces blood levels of vitamin B_5 and lowers absorption of the nutrient by the intestines. Also, alcoholics tend to substitute alcohol—which has no real nutritional value—for nutrient-dense foods, so they generally don't take in adequate amounts of vitamin B_5 and other nutrients.

❏ *Is your diet high in processed foods?* Significant amounts of pantothenic acid are lost in foods when they are milled, canned, frozen, cooked, or otherwise processed.

ing foot syndrome." Symptoms improved when the prisoners were given pantothenic acid; supplementation with other B vitamins did not bring about a positive response. However, the men were severely malnourished and deficient in *all* of the essential vitamins, not just in the B vitamins. So while burning foot syndrome seemed to get better with adequate pantothenic acid intake, studies were never conducted to conclusively determine if B_5 deficiency was indeed responsible for the illness.

The most common symptoms caused by long-term pantothenic acid deficiency are headaches, nausea, abdominal cramps, fatigue, depression, increased susceptibility to colds, insomnia, and numbness and tingling in the hands and feet.

TOXICITY SYMPTOMS

The human body excretes excess pantothenic acid in urine. Not surprisingly, then, serious toxicity symptoms have not been reported. Very high doses of B_5—10 grams or more per day—may cause diarrhea or water retention. Intake at these excessive levels is not recommended.

OPTIMAL DAILY ALLOWANCE

Although a formal RDA has not been established for pantothenic acid, some studies indicate that daily doses of at least 10 milligrams are sufficient to meet the needs of adults, including women who are pregnant or breast-feeding. The recommended Optimal Daily Allowance of pantothenic acid for all adults ranges from 10 to 100 milligrams. The higher levels are appropriate during times of prolonged stress, and for people who regularly engage in vigorous exercise.

Food Sources

As mentioned earlier, most foods contain at least small amounts of pantothenic acid. Some of the best sources of the nutrient are potatoes, saltwater fish, pork, beef, milk, organ meats, salmon, legumes, whole-grain cereals, eggs, yeast, and fresh vegetables. It's important to note that a large percentage of the B_5 contained in foods may be lost due to food processing, such as milling, canning, cooking, and freezing.

Are You Maximizing Your Vitamin B₅ Intake?

Studies have shown that most people in the United States consume 5 to 10 milligrams of vitamin B₅ daily from dietary sources—a level at or somewhat below the minimum Optimal Daily Allowance. While it is possible to reach this minimum through diet alone, it's difficult to achieve higher intakes without relying on vitamin B₅ supplements. Where do you stand?

You can use the information in Table 12.1 to determine your average daily intake of vitamin B₅. The foods and beverages included in this table are arranged according to the percentage of the Optimal Daily Allowance of vitamin B₅ they contain. Remember, the ODA of pantothenic acid is 10 to 100 milligrams daily. For this self-test, we'll use the lowest ODA in the range, 10 milligrams.

Start by keeping a food diary for at least three to four days; the longer you keep the diary, the more accurate your calculations will be. Write down everything you eat and drink, as well as the estimated serving size, and refer to the table on page 129 to determine the percentage of the ODA that each food or beverage provides. At the end of each day, add up all of the percentages to see if you've reached 100 percent for the day. (If your ODA falls on the higher end of the range, take this into account when you calculate your percentages.)

If you find that, on average, you do not take in 100 percent of your ODA for vitamin B₅, then you may decide that you want to take vitamin supplements for optimal health. But how much of this nutrient do you need to take to reach your ODA? Here's an example of how to perform this calculation: Let's say you determine that you are getting 60 percent (0.60) of your target intake through diet alone. Multiply 0.60 and 10 milligrams (the ODA of pantothenic acid) and you'll find that you're consuming 6 milligrams of pantothenic acid in your diet. To make up the difference, then, you should take in 4 milligrams of pantothenic acid in supplement form. Most multivitamins contain at least the minimum ODA of pantothenic acid, and often more—so if you take a multivitamin tablet each day, you're probably getting all you need.

Table 12.1. Percent of Vitamin B_5 ODA in Common Foods and Beverages

Food	Serving Size	Food	Serving Size
5 Percent		Sweet potato, baked	1 medium
Acorn squash, baked	½ cup	Tomato juice , canned	6 ounces
Avocado, California	½ medium	**10 Percent**	
Beef, top round, broiled	3½ ounces	Avocado, Florida	½ medium
Black-eyed peas, boiled	1 cup	Chicken, dark and	
Buttermilk	1 cup	light meat, roasted	3½ ounces
		leg meat, roasted	1 leg
Chicken, thigh meat, roasted	1 thigh	Egg	1 large
Corn, yellow, boiled	½ cup	Figs, dried	10 figs
Cottage cheese, low-fat	1 cup	Lentils, boiled	1 cup
Dates, dried	10 dates	Lima beans, boiled	1 cup
Garbanzo beans, boiled	1 cup	Milk, 1%	1 cup
Great Northern beans, boiled	1 cup	Mushrooms	½ cup
		Peanuts	1 ounce
Herring	3 ounces	Potato, baked, with or without skin	1 medium
Hubbard squash, baked	½ cup	Turkey, dark and light meat, roasted	3½ ounces
Ice cream, vanilla	1 cup		
Ice milk, vanilla	1 cup	**15 Percent**	
Navy beans, boiled	1 cup	Salmon	3 ounces
Parsnips, boiled	½ cup	Trout	3 ounces
Pecans	1 ounce	Yogurt, low-fat	8 ounces
Pinto beans, boiled	1 cup	**50 Percent**	
Pork		Beef liver, braised	3½ ounces
loin, roasted	3½ ounces	**55 Percent**	
shoulder, roasted	3½ ounces		
Strawberries	1 cup	Chicken liver, simmered	3½ ounces

RECOMMENDATIONS

When it comes to nutrition, there's a lot of important information to remember—so it helps to have what you need to know right at your fingertips. The most critical facts about pantothenic acid are summarized below.

What is the Optimal Daily Allowance of pantothenic acid?
The ODA of pantothenic acid for men and women ranges from 10 to 100 milligrams.

What circumstances might affect the amount of pantothenic acid you need to take in each day?
Some lifestyle factors can affect the amount of vitamin B5 you consume or decrease the amount that your body is able to absorb and use. You'll have to be particularly conscientious about taking in the ODA of vitamin B5 if you have diabetes. Eating a diet that includes a lot of processed foods or drinking large amounts of alcohol also increases the risk of vitamin B5 deficiency, so you should be careful to take in your optimal allowance.

Is it possible to consume the optimal amount of pantothenic acid through diet alone?
Because vitamin B5 is found in so many foods, it is certainly possible to take in the minimum ODA from dietary sources alone. However, achieving a higher intake level (15 milligrams or more) is difficult if you don't also take supplements.

Chapter 13

Vitamin B$_6$ (Pyridoxine)

Vitamin B$_6$ was first identified and described in the late-1930s. The discovery of this nutrient actually grew out of research aimed at isolating other nutrients. In fact, vitamin B$_6$ was initially thought to be the pellagra-preventive factor present in some foods, prior to the discovery of vitamin B$_3$. As it turns out, vitamin B$_6$ does not prevent pellagra; however, the nutrient is now known to take part in over 100 enzymatic processes. It is involved in the metabolism of amino acids, which the body uses to build proteins necessary for growth and repair of all body structures. Vitamin B$_6$ is also essential to the proper functioning of the central nervous system, and it promotes healthy blood and blood vessels. And that's only part of the long list of ways in which vitamin B$_6$ functions to keep the body strong!

In 1942, scientists discovered that vitamin B$_6$ exists naturally in three closely related forms: *pyridoxine, pyridoxal,* and *pyridoxamine.* The pyridoxine form of vitamin B$_6$ is usually found in plants and seeds, while pyridoxal and pyridoxamine are present mostly in animal products. Nutritional supplements generally contain pyridoxine.

FUNCTIONS IN THE BODY

Vitamin B$_6$ is involved in many body processes. It functions as a coenzyme that aids in the metabolism of protein from food. For example, the vitamin assists in the body's transamination processes, in which an amino group is transferred from an abundant amino acid to a different molecule, usually to produce an amino acid that the body needs in greater amounts. Vitamin B_6 also aids in the body's conversion of the amino acid tryptophan to vitamin B_3, or niacin. (See page 117.)

Another vital function of vitamin B_6 is its role in the formation of hemoglobin, the substance in red blood cells that carries oxygen. In addition, B_6 is an important factor in the synthesis of red blood cells and of infection-fighting immune cells called antibodies.

Proper functioning of the central nervous system depends upon adequate vitamin B_6 intake, because the nutrient is necessary for the production of neurotransmitters in the brain. Neurotransmitters are chemical carriers in the brain that help transmit impulses along nerve cells.

Vitamin B_6 is also considered to be an energy-yielding nutrient. It assists in the breakdown of glycogen—a storage form of energy in the body—into glucose (sugar) molecules, which are the body's primary source of usable energy. The nutrient also plays a role in the utilization of fats for energy.

HEALTH BENEFITS

If you've read the ads in health magazines, you may have seen claims that large doses of B_6 can alleviate depression, premenstrual syndrome (PMS), asthma, muscle fatigue, and even autism. However, more research needs to be conducted in these areas before experts can positively state that the vitamin provides these benefits.

Scientific evidence has shown that vitamin B_6 may be useful in the prevention of coronary heart disease because it helps to reduce blood levels of the amino acid *homocysteine*. High levels of homocysteine in the blood have been associated with damage to the artery walls and atherosclerosis.

Nearly thirty years ago, a Harvard University researcher implicated high blood levels of homocysteine as a risk factor for atherosclerosis and coronary heart disease. This theory gained tremendous support recently, due to a study conducted at Harvard University's medical school, in which researchers monitored the health of thousands of physicians for many years. The results of the study showed that doctors who had high levels of homocys-

Are You at Risk of Vitamin B_6 Deficiency?

How do you know if you're at risk of vitamin B_6 deficiency? Take a moment to review the questions below. If you answer yes to any of these questions, you have an above-average risk of developing a deficiency.

❑ *Do you regularly take any of the following medications: isoniazid, hydralazine, or penicillamine?* Isoniazid, which is used to treat tuberculosis; hydralazine, used for high blood pressure; and penicillamine, which is taken by patients with rheumatoid arthritis, all increase the excretion of vitamin B_6 in the urine.

❑ *Do you take oral contraceptives?* Birth control pills have been conclusively proven to alter concentrations of nutrients in the blood. Blood levels of vitamin B_6 can decrease by as much as 15 to 20 percent in women who use oral contraceptives.

❑ *Do you drink large amounts of alcohol?* Alcohol can destroy vitamin B_6, dramatically decreasing blood levels of the nutrient. Therefore, the more alcohol you drink, the more likely you are to experience vitamin B_6 deficiency. Obviously, this effect has the greatest impact on alcoholics and, in fact, some 20 to 30 percent of alcoholics are deficient in vitamin B_6. Also, alcoholics tend to substitute alcohol—which has no real nutritional value—for nutrient-dense foods, so they generally don't take in adequate amounts of vitamin B_6 and other nutrients.

❑ *Is your diet high in protein?* Vitamin B_6 is required for protein metabolism, so the more protein you consume, the more vitamin B_6 your body needs.

❑ *Are you pregnant or breast-feeding?* Pregnancy is a time of increased nutritional needs because the growth of a new person requires every known nutrient. Women who are breast-feeding can lose as much as 0.25 milligrams of this vitamin per liter of breast milk. The ODA of vitamin B_6 is more than adequate to meet the increased needs of women who are pregnant or breast-feeding.

teine were three times more likely to suffer heart attacks than those with low blood levels of the amino acid. This means that high homocysteine ranks as a key risk factor for coronary heart disease, sharing the spotlight with other known risks such as smoking and high cholesterol.

It is now widely accepted that inadequate amounts of vitamin B_6—along with the B vitamins folic acid and vitamin B_{12}—are likely to lead to high levels of homocysteine. Because of the link between high homocysteine levels and coronary heart disease evidenced in the Physician's Study, many doctors now recommend supplementation with these B vitamins to help protect against coronary heart disease.

DEFICIENCY SYMPTOMS

Vitamin B_6 deficiencies are rare, thanks to the wide availability of this nutrient in everyday foods. Deficiency is often recognized by the manifestation of skin disorders, such as scaling of the skin. Inflammation of the tongue and mucous membranes of the mouth may also occur. Other symptoms include depression, irritability, dizziness, and weakness, as well as convulsions, which most frequently occur in infants. Additional symptoms include anemia, weakened immune function, and nausea and vomiting.

TOXICITY SYMPTOMS

Isolated case reports have shown that as few as 200 milligrams daily of vitamin B_6 can cause neurological problems, including numbness in the hands and feet, and difficulty walking. However, the nutrient is generally safe for most people in doses of up to 500 milligrams daily. Warning signs of toxicity may become apparent when amounts greater than 500 milligrams are consumed. These symptoms include dermatitis—or skin rash—related to sun exposure, difficulty walking, and numbness or tingling in the hands and feet. However, these adverse effects usually disappear when high doses are discontinued. Doses of 2,000 milligrams or more daily have been associated with permanent nerve damage.

OPTIMAL DAILY ALLOWANCE

The recommended Optimal Daily Allowance of vitamin B_6 is 4 to 10 milligrams. This range is appropriate for men and women.

In determining your optimal vitamin B_6 intake, keep in mind that your requirement varies according to different circumstances in your life. For example, if you're at risk of developing atherosclerosis and coronary heart disease due to high blood levels of homocysteine, you'll want to make sure you're taking in levels of vitamin B_6 from the higher end of the ODA range suggested above.

Food Sources

Vitamin B_6 is present in a wide variety of foods, although many contain low levels of the nutrient. The richest sources of vitamin B_6 include beef, brewer's yeast, eggs, fish, liver, peanuts, peas, pork, poultry, soybeans, spinach, walnuts, and wheat germ. Dairy products and most vegetables and fruits contain relatively little B_6.

The vitamin B_6 content of foods is altered by cooking, food processing and refining, and heat, oxygen, and light.

Are You Maximizing Your Vitamin B_6 Intake?

It's possible to reach the Optimal Daily Allowance of vitamin B_6 through dietary sources alone, but research has shown that most Americans fail to meet even the RDA for this vitamin. In 1994, government surveys found that men consume an average of 2.23 milligrams of B_6 daily, while women consume an average of 1.51 milligrams. As you can surmise, most people need to supplement with vitamin B_6 to reach the minimum ODA of 4 milligrams, and individuals who are aiming for the higher end of the range will definitely benefit from supplementation. Where do you stand?

You can use the information in Table 13.1 to determine your average daily intake of vitamin B_6. The foods and beverages included in this table are arranged according to the percentage of the Optimal Daily Allowance of vitamin B_6 they contain. Remember, the ODA of vitamin B_6 ranges from 4 to 10 milligrams. For this self-test, we'll use the lowest ODA in the range, 4 milligrams.

Start by keeping an accurate food diary for at least three to four days; the longer you keep the diary, the more accurate your calculations will be. Write down everything you eat and drink, as well as the estimated serving size, and refer to the table on page 136 to determine the percentage of the ODA that each food or beverage

Table 13.1. Percent of Vitamin B$_6$ ODA in Common Foods and Beverages

Food	Serving Size	Food	Serving Size
5 Percent		Swordfish	3 ounces
Acorn squash, baked	1/2 cup	Tuna, canned in water	3 ounces
Avocado, California	1/2 medium	Tomato juice, canned	6 ounces
Beef		Wheat germ, toasted	1/4 cup
bottom round, braised	3 1/2 ounces	**10 Percent**	
brisket, braised	3 1/2 ounces		
flank steak, broiled	3 1/2 ounces	Avocado, Florida	1 medium
ground (lean), baked	3 1/2 ounces	Banana	1 medium
Chicken, leg meat, roasted	1 leg	Beef, top round, braised	3 1/2 ounces
Cod	3 ounces	Bran Flakes cereal	1 ounce
Garbanzo beans, boiled	1 cup	Carrot juice, canned	6 ounces
Great Northern beans, boiled	1 cup	Chicken	
		breast meat, roasted	1/2 breast
Haddock	3 ounces	dark and light meat,	
Halibut	3 ounces	roasted	3 1/2 ounces
		liver, simmered	3 1/2 ounces
Herring	3 ounces	Corn Flakes cereal	1 ounce
Kidney beans, boiled	1 cup	Cream of Wheat,	
Lentils, boiled	1 cup	instant	1 packet
Lima beans, boiled	1 cup	Figs, dried	10 figs
Mackerel	3 ounces	Ham, canned	3 1/2 ounces
Manhattan clam chowder	1 cup	Oatmeal, instant	1 packet
		Potato, baked, with skin	1 medium
Miso	1/2 cup	Raisin Bran cereal	1 ounce
Navy beans, boiled	1 cup	Salmon	3 ounces
Pineapple juice, canned	1 cup	Turkey, dark and	
Pinto beans, boiled	1 cup	light meat, roasted	3 1/2 ounces
Pork		**20 Percent**	
loin, roasted	3 1/2 ounces	Beef liver, braised	3 1/2 ounces
shoulder, roasted	3 1/2 ounces	**50 Percent**	
Prunes, dried	10 prunes	Product 19 cereal	1 ounce
Raisins, golden, seedless	2/3 cup	Total cereal	1 ounce
Sweet potato, baked	1 medium		

provides. (If your optimal dose falls elsewhere in our recommended range, take that into account when calculating percentages.) At the end of the day, add up all of the percentages to see if you've reached 100 percent for the day.

If you find that, on average, you do not take in 100 percent of your ODA for vitamin B_6, then you may decide that you want to take vitamin supplements for optimal health. But how much of this nutrient do you need to take to reach your ODA? Here's an example of how to perform this calculation: Let's say you determine that you are getting 25 percent (0.25) of your vitamin B_6 target intake through diet alone. Multiply 0.25 and 4 milligrams (the ODA of vitamin B_6), and you'll find that you're consuming 1 milligram of vitamin B_6 in your diet. To make up the difference, then, you should take in 3 milligrams of vitamin B_6 in supplement form.

RECOMMENDATIONS

When it comes to nutrition, there's a lot of important information to remember—so it helps to have what you need to know right at your fingertips. The most critical facts about vitamin B_6 are summarized below.

What is the Optimal Daily Allowance of vitamin B_6?
The ODA of vitamin B_6 for men and women is 4 to 10 milligrams. It's especially important to aim for the higher intakes in the ODA range if you are at risk of cardiovascular disease.

What circumstances might affect the amount of vitamin B_6 you need to take in each day?
Some lifestyle factors can affect the amount of vitamin B_6 you consume or decrease the amount that your body is able to absorb and use. You'll have to be particularly conscientious about taking in the ODA of vitamin B_6 if:

- You take certain medications, including isoniazid, hydralazine, or penicillamine.

- You use oral contraceptives.

- You drink large amounts of alcohol.

- You eat a high-protein diet.

- You are pregnant or breast-feeding.

Is it possible to consume the optimal amount of vitamin B_6 through diet alone?

Chances are, most Americans don't take in the RDA of vitamin B_6, much less the ODA. Therefore, it seems that many of us would benefit from taking supplemental B_6.

Chapter 14

Vitamin B$_{12}$ (Cobalamin)

Vitamin B$_{12}$, or cobalamin, is most often associated with the prevention of a severe form of anemia known as *pernicious anemia*. Anemia is a reduction in either the number of red blood cells or the amount of hemoglobin in the blood. The pernicious form of anemia was so labeled because of its devastating and lasting effects, including nerve damage and paralysis.

FUNCTIONS IN THE BODY

Vitamin B$_{12}$ is necessary for the manufacture of red blood cells, which are responsible for transporting oxygen to all of the body's cells. It also helps maintain the fatty tissue known as the *myelin sheath* that surrounds and protects nerve cells. As such, the vitamin plays an important part in healthy nervous system function.

Additionally, vitamin B$_{12}$ is involved in the synthesis of protein; the metabolism of carbohydrates and fats; the body's use of folic acid; and the synthesis of DNA and RNA, the genetic materials that are necessary for cell replication and development.

HEALTH BENEFITS

Vitamin B$_{12}$ plays a part in preventing cardiovascular disease by helping to reduce blood levels of the amino acid homocysteine. High homocysteine levels have been associated with the buildup of plaque along the inside walls of the arteries, increasing the risk

The History of Vitamin B₁₂

Pernicious anemia ravaged the populations of Europe during the nineteenth century. Although the cause was not then apparent, the symptoms of the condition were merciless—diarrhea and sore tongue in the early stages; nerve damage and severe mental disturbance as the condition progressed; and, in the worst cases, death. Under the pressures of trying to understand the potentially life-threatening disease, researchers frantically searched for answers. But the idea that the disease could be caused by a nutritional deficit was never put forth. To the contrary, individuals affected by pernicious anemia appeared to be well-nourished.

Finally, in the 1920s and 1930s, Nobel Prize-winning experimenters George Minot and William Murphy discovered clues to the disease. They demonstrated that patients who ate liver had a greater chance of recovering from this form of anemia. By the late 1940s, vitamin B_{12} was isolated and identified as the substance that was so successful in overcoming the killer disease. Today, we know that liver is one of the richest sources of vitamin B_{12}.

---

of angina, heart attack, and stroke. Recently, scientists have discovered that vitamin B_{12}, vitamin B_6, and folic acid are all important factors in the breakdown of homocysteine in the body, keeping the amino acid from building up to toxic levels and accumulating in the arteries. Supplementation with these B vitamins may help normalize homocysteine levels, thereby reducing the risk of cardiovascular disease.

In 1993, researchers in South Africa conducted a study involving thirty men with high blood levels of homocysteine and correspondingly low levels of vitamin B_{12}. The participants received varying amounts of B_{12} (as well as other B vitamins) or supplements of beta-carotene. Six weeks later, the researchers again measured the participants' blood levels of homocysteine. The results showed that the men taking B vitamin supplements had normal homocysteine levels, which reduced their risk of developing cardiovascular disease. On the other hand, the men taking beta-carotene still had elevated homocysteine levels, and were thus at a greater risk of developing cardiovascular disease.

DEFICIENCY SYMPTOMS

Vitamin B$_{12}$ deficiency is most commonly associated with pernicious anemia, a condition that is characterized by weakness and fatigue, weight loss, diarrhea, sore tongue, and pale skin. Severe deficiency can cause impaired nervous system function and even permanent nerve damage. Psychological disturbances, including moodiness and depression, are also warning signs of vitamin B$_{12}$ deficiency.

Unfortunately, adequate intake of vitamin B$_{12}$ does not necessarily protect against B$_{12}$ deficiency. The body's absorption of vitamin B$_{12}$ from food and supplements requires the assistance of a protein called *intrinsic factor,* which is produced by cells in the stomach lining. The intrinsic factor attaches to the vitamin, and carries it into the digestive tract, where it can be absorbed into the bloodstream. Because of a genetic defect, or due to injury to the stomach, some individuals cannot produce enough of this factor, and so they cannot absorb vitamin B$_{12}$.

In some cases, vitamin B$_{12}$ deficiency is misdiagnosed as folic acid deficiency because the body needs vitamin B$_{12}$ in order to process and use folic acid. If the prescribed treatment is folic acid supplementation, then the B$_{12}$ deficiency will only worsen. Plus, the body won't be able to put the extra folic acid to good use unless adequate vitamin B$_{12}$ is present.

TOXICITY SYMPTOMS

Toxicity symptoms have not been associated with vitamin B$_{12}$ consumption, even when the nutrient is taken in high doses.

OPTIMAL DAILY ALLOWANCE

Until recently, the Optimal Daily Allowance of vitamin B$_{12}$ was 5 micrograms. However, because we are now aware of the important role the nutrient plays in controlling blood levels of the amino acid homocysteine, it makes a great deal of sense to raise the suggested intake. The current ODA of vitamin B$_{12}$ is 100 to 400 micrograms per day. Although this is many times higher than the RDA, the new recommendation is warranted due to the proven link between

Are You at Risk of Vitamin B$_{12}$ Deficiency?

How do you know if you're at risk of vitamin B$_{12}$ deficiency? Take a moment to review the questions below. If you answer yes to any of these questions, you have an above-average risk of developing a deficiency.

❑ *Do you take any of the following medications: colchicine, cholesytramine, or omeprazole?* Experts warn that colchicine, which is used to treat gout; cholestyramine, a cholesterol-lowering agent; and omeprazole, used in the treatment of ulcers, have all been shown to interfere with the absorption of vitamin B$_{12}$. The antibiotic neomycin also appears to lower B$_{12}$ levels.

❑ *Have you suffered a stomach injury?* Injury to or removal of any part of the stomach can reduce the production of intrinsic factor, leading to impaired vitamin B$_{12}$ absorption.

❑ *Are you a strict vegetarian?* Vitamin B$_{12}$ exists naturally only in animal products, not in plants. If you do not eat animal foods, and you do not take in vitamin B$_{12}$ from fortified foods or vitamin supplements, then you may be at risk of deficiency. Children on vegetarian diets are particularly susceptible to B$_{12}$ deficiencies because they have not yet built up adequate stores of the vitamin.

❑ *Do you prepare the majority of your food in a microwave oven?* Microwaves can decrease vitamin B$_{12}$ activity by up to 40 percent.

❑ *Are you pregnant or breast-feeding?* Pregnancy is a time of increased nutritional needs because the growth of a new person requires every known nutrient. Since vitamin B$_{12}$ is so important in the manufacture of new cells, a growing fetus needs 0.1 to 0.2 micrograms of the nutrient daily from the expectant mother's intake in order to develop properly. Women who are breast-feeding should increase their vitamin B$_{12}$ intake to compensate for the 0.6 micrograms that is contained in every liter of breast milk. The ODA of vitamin B$_{12}$ is more than adequate to meet the increased needs of women who are pregnant or breast-feeding.

❑ *Are you an older person?* With increasing age, the body produces smaller amounts of the intrinsic factor that is necessary for B$_{12}$ absorption. Therefore, older adults often have more trouble absorbing B$_{12}$ than do younger people.

high homocysteine levels and the increased risk of cardiovascular disease.

Food Sources

Animal foods are the only natural sources of vitamin B$_{12}$. The richest sources of this nutrient are organ meats (kidney and liver), fish, clams, poultry, beef, milk, cheese, and egg yolks. If you are a strict vegetarian who does not eat any animal foods, vitamin B$_{12}$ supplements are probably your best bet to get the amounts you need. Soybean milk substitutes and fortified breakfast cereals are usually good choices for all vegetarians.

Vitamin B$_{12}$ is relatively stable when exposed to light and heat, and only small amounts of the nutrient are lost in cooking.

Are You Maximizing Your Vitamin B$_{12}$ Intake?

Nutritional surveys have shown that, on average, American men take in about 6 micrograms of vitamin B$_{12}$ daily, while women come close to 5 micrograms. These amounts are far below the Optimal Daily Allowance of vitamin B$_{12}$. Clearly, most men and women in the United States will benefit from supplementation with this vitamin. Where do you stand?

You can use the information in Table 14.1 to determine your average daily intake of vitamin B$_{12}$. The foods and beverages included in this table are arranged according to the percentage of the Optimal Daily Allowance of vitamin B$_{12}$ they contain. Remember, the ODA of vitamin B$_{12}$ is 100 to 400 micrograms per day. For this self-test, we'll use the lowest ODA in the range, 100 micrograms.

Start by keeping a food diary for at least three to four days; the longer you keep the diary, the more accurate your calculations will be. Write down everything you eat and drink, as well as the estimated serving size, and refer to the table on page 144 to determine the percentage of the ODA that each food or beverage provides. At the end of the day, add up all of the percentages to see if you've reached 100 percent for the day.

If you find that, on average, you do not take in 100 percent of your ODA for vitamin B$_{12}$, then you may decide that you want to take vitamin supplements for optimal health. But how much of

Table 14.1. Percent of Vitamin B$_{12}$ ODA in Common Foods and Beverages			
Food	**Serving Size**	**Food**	**Serving Size**
5 Percent		Oysters	6 medium
Crab, cooked	3 ounces	**20 Percent**	
Mackerel	3 ounces	Chicken liver, simmered	3$\frac{1}{2}$ ounces
Manhattan clam chowder	1 cup	**40 Percent**	
		Clams	4 large or 9 small
Trout	3 ounces		
10 Percent		**70 Percent**	
Herring	3 ounces	Beef liver, braised	3$\frac{1}{2}$ ounces

this nutrient do you need to take to reach your ODA? Here's an example of how to perform this calculation: Let's say that you determine that you are getting 80 percent (0.80) of your vitamin B$_{12}$ target intake through diet alone. Multiply 0.80 and 100 micrograms (the ODA of vitamin B$_{12}$), and you'll find that you're consuming 80 micrograms of B$_{12}$ in your diet. To make up the difference, then, you should take in 20 micrograms of vitamin B$_{12}$ in supplement form.

RECOMMENDATIONS

When it comes to nutrition, there's a lot of important information to remember—so it helps to have what you need to know right at your fingertips. The most critical facts about vitamin B$_{12}$ are summarized below.

What is the Optimal Daily Allowance of vitamin B$_{12}$?
The ODA of vitamin B$_{12}$ for men and women ranges from 100 to 400 micrograms.

What circumstances might affect the amount of vitamin B$_{12}$ you need to take in each day?
Some lifestyle or health factors can affect the amount of vitamin B$_{12}$ you consume or decrease the amount that your body is able to absorb and use. You'll have to be particularly conscientious about taking in the ODA of vitamin B$_{12}$ if:

- You take certain medications, including colchicine, cholestyramine, or omeprazole.

- You have suffered a stomach injury.

- You are a strict vegetarian.

- You prepare the majority of your food in a microwave oven.

- You are pregnant or breast-feeding.

- You are an older person.

Is it possible to consume the optimal amount of vitamin B$_{12}$ through diet alone?

Unless you eat dozens of clams, lots of liver, or entire boxes of fortified cereal every day, you're probably not meeting your ODA of vitamin B$_{12}$ through dietary sources alone. Indeed, surveys have shown that, on average, American men and women take in amounts far below the Optimal Daily Allowance. So while it's still a good idea to choose foods rich in vitamin B$_{12}$, it's likely that you'll have to rely on a supplement to reach the ODA.

Chapter 15

Biotin

Biotin gets its name from the Greek word *bios,* meaning "life." As with vitamin K, biotin can be produced by bacteria in the intestinal tract—in fact, our bodies often produce enough of this B vitamin to meet our daily requirements. However, this nutrient is also found in food sources, most notably organ meats.

FUNCTIONS IN THE BODY

Like the other members of the B complex family, biotin is important for the metabolism of carbohydrates, fats, and proteins for energy.

HEALTH BENEFITS

Biotin has few substantiated uses as a treatment for medical conditions. Its medicinal use seems to be limited to the treatment of *seborrheic dermatitis,* which is characterized by scaly patches of skin that result from a disorder of oil-secreting glands called sebaceous glands. This condition most often occurs in infants.

DEFICIENCY SYMPTOMS

Because biotin is manufactured by the body and is also found in food sources, deficiencies of this nutrient are rare. Deficiency symptoms include dry, scaly skin and dermatitis, loss of appetite, muscle pain, nausea and vomiting, and neurological problems such as insomnia or depression.

Are You at Risk of Biotin Deficiency?

How do you know if you're at risk of biotin deficiency? Take a moment to review the questions below. If you answer yes to any of these questions, you have an above-average risk of developing a deficiency.

❏ *Do you take anticonvulsant medications?* Anticonvulsants, including phenytoin, phenobarbital, and carbamazepine, interfere with biotin's activity in the body.

❏ *Are raw egg whites a regular part of your diet?* Egg whites contain an indigestible protein called *avidin* that interferes with the body's absorption of biotin. This can easily be remedied, however—cooking eggs will destroy avidin.

❏ *Are you pregnant or breast-feeding?* Pregnancy is a time of increased nutritional needs because the growth of a new person requires every known nutrient. Women who are breast-feeding also need extra biotin to compensate for the amount that is contained in breast milk. The ODA of biotin is more than adequate to meet the increased needs of women who are pregnant or breast-feeding.

TOXICITY SYMPTOMS

Toxicity has not been reported with biotin, even at doses as high as 10 milligrams per day.

OPTIMAL DAILY ALLOWANCE

The ODA of biotin for men and women ranges from 30 to 100 micrograms, which is safe and sufficient to meet the needs of all healthy adults.

Food Sources

The best sources of biotin include organ meats such as liver; some dairy products, including milk and cheese; brewer's yeast and other nutritional yeasts; soybeans and soy flour; egg yolks; fish; nuts; and cheese.

Biotin is a stable nutrient, and so is not destroyed during cooking.

Are You Maximizing Your Biotin Intake?

Few studies have been done on biotin consumption in the United States. According to one report, average biotin intake among men and women reaches from 28 to 42 micrograms per day—the low end of the ODA range. Individuals who are aiming for the higher intakes from the suggested range will probably benefit from supplementation. Where do you stand?

You can use the information in Table 15.1 to determine your average daily intake of biotin. The foods and beverages included in this table are arranged according to the percentage of the Optimal Daily Allowance of biotin they contain. Remember, the ODA of biotin ranges from 30 to 100 micrograms. For this self-test, we'll use the lowest ODA in the range, 30 micrograms.

Start by keeping a food diary for at least three to four days; the longer you keep the diary, the more accurate your calculations will be. Write down everything you eat and drink, as well as the estimated serving size, and refer to the table on page 150 to determine the percentage of the ODA that each food or beverage provides. (If your optimal dose falls elsewhere in the recommended range, take that into account when calculating percentages.) At the end of each day, add up all of the percentages to see if you've reached 100 percent for the day.

If you find that, on average, you do not take in 100 percent of your ODA for biotin, then you may decide that you want to take vitamin supplements for optimal health. But how much of this nutrient do you need to take to reach your ODA? Here's an example of how to perform this calculation: Let's say you determine that you are getting only 50 percent (0.50) of your target intake through diet alone. Multiply 0.50 and 30 micrograms (the ODA of biotin), and you'll find that you are consuming 15 micrograms of biotin in your diet. To make up the difference, then, you should take in 15 micrograms of biotin in supplement form.

RECOMMENDATIONS

When it comes to nutrition, there's a lot of important information to remember—so it helps to have what you need to know right at your fingertips. The most critical facts about biotin are summarized below.

Table 15.1. Percent of Biotin ODA in Common Foods and Beverages

Food	Serving Size	Food	Serving Size
5 Percent		**20 Percent**	
Haddock, steamed	3 ounces	Hazelnuts	1 ounce
Herring, grilled	3 ounces	Oatmeal	$1/2$ cup
Mackerel, fried	3 ounces	Peanuts	1 ounce
Walnuts	1 ounce	**40 Percent**	
Yogurt, low-fat	8 ounces	Beef liver	3 ounces
10 Percent		**100 Percent**	
Egg	1 large	Chicken liver	3 ounces
Peanut butter	1 tablespoon		

What is the Optimal Daily Allowance of biotin?
The ODA of biotin for men and women ranges from 30 to 100 micrograms.

What circumstances might affect the amount of biotin you need to take in each day?
Some lifestyle or health factors can affect the amount of biotin you consume or decrease the amount that your body is able to absorb and use. You'll have to be particularly conscientious about taking in the ODA of biotin if you take anticonvulsant medications, including phenytoin, phenobarbital, and carbamazepine, or if you are pregnant or breast-feeding. Also, if raw egg whites are a regular part of your diet, be sure to take in your optimal allowance of biotin, since egg whites can interfere with the absorption of this vitamin.

Is it possible to consume the optimal amount of biotin through diet alone?
Research shows that the average American does manage to reach (or comes close to reaching) the lower end of the ODA range for biotin. However, people who are aiming for the higher intakes from the suggested range will probably benefit from supplementation.

Chapter 16

Folic Acid

Although the B vitamin folic acid—also called folate or folacin—was first identified in the 1940s, it's only lately that the nutrient has been getting a lot of attention. In the 1990s, researchers discovered that folic acid has some very important health benefits. For one thing, it can protect against *neural tube defects* (NTDs), severe birth abnormalities that affect the brain and spine. Another reason for folic acid's recent popularity is the discovery that, along with vitamins B_6 and B_{12}, this B vitamin plays an important role in reducing homocysteine levels, which means that it helps protect against coronary heart disease.

FUNCTIONS IN THE BODY

Folic acid and vitamin B_{12} are important for the metabolism of amino acids and the synthesis of proteins. These B vitamins are also involved in the synthesis of DNA and RNA, which are the genetic materials contained in all cells. The nucleic acids are necessary for cell division and cell replication, and are therefore essential to tissue growth. Additionally, research has shown that folic acid protects against defects of the neural tube, the structure in the embryo that gives rise to the central nervous system. For this reason, expectant mothers need extra folic acid during pregnancy. The U.S. Public Health Service and the American Academy of Pediatrics now advise all women of childbearing age to take in at least 0.4 milligrams (400 micrograms) of folic acid daily in order to reduce the risk of neural tube defects in newborns.

Folic acid has also been shown to help prevent coronary heart disease. It is one of a trio of vitamins—the others are vitamins B_6 and B_{12}—that break down homocysteine in the body. In the early 1970s, a Harvard University researcher implicated high blood levels of homocysteine as a cause of atherosclerosis and coronary heart disease—a risk factor that affects nearly 20 percent of the population. Vitamin B_6, vitamin B_{12}, and folic acid assist liver enzymes in degrading homocysteine, thereby decreasing its levels in the blood.

With the help of vitamin B_{12}, folic acid also ensures the proper formation of red blood cells. A deficiency of either one of these vitamins can cause a form of anemia that is characterized by large, immature red blood cells.

HEALTH BENEFITS

Some of the most exciting news in vitamin research comes from studies of the connection between folic acid and the prevention of birth defects and cardiovascular disease.

Neural Tube Defects

Statistics show that about 2,500 babies with neural tube defects (NTDs) are born each year in the United States; worldwide, the number reaches 300,000 to 400,000 cases. Some examples of NTDs include *spina bifida* and *anencephaly*. Spina bifida is a condition in which one or more vertebrae do not develop completely, leaving part of the spinal cord unprotected. The severity of symptoms varies; some children do not appear to be affected, while others may be weak or paralyzed in areas associated with the damaged part of the spinal cord. Anencephaly is a birth defect in which most or all of the infant's brain is missing because it does not develop. An infant with this condition cannot survive, and is either stillborn or dies shortly after birth. Although researchers suspected for some time that vitamins may offer a protective effect against neural tube defects, the most convincing evidence now relates specifically to folic acid.

A seven-country study, published in 1991, examined the effects of several different vitamins on the occurrence of neural tube defects. The study involved 1,817 women who had conceived a child with an NTD. The women were divided into four groups: One group supplemented with 4 milligrams of folic acid daily; women in the next group took other vitamins; another group supplemented with 4 milligrams of folic acid daily, along with other vitamins; and the last group of women took a placebo, with no active ingredients. The results showed that women taking 4 milligrams per day of folic acid—with or without other vitamins—reduced their chances of another NTD pregnancy by 72 percent. In contrast, participants taking multivitamin supplements without folic acid, as well as those taking the placebo, did not reduce their risk of another NTD pregnancy. The researchers who conducted this study advised that "public health measures should be taken to ensure that the diet of all women who may bear children contains an adequate amount of folic acid."

In 1992, Hungarian researchers published a report of their study on nutrient supplementation and pregnancy. This study involved 7,500 women who were planning to become pregnant, most for the first time. At least one month before they became pregnant, one group of women began taking a multivitamin containing 0.8 milligrams of folic acid, plus eleven other vitamins, four minerals, and three trace elements; within the same time frame, the other group started taking supplements of only trace elements. All of the participants continued taking their supplements after conception until at least the second missed menstrual period. More than 4,000 of the women involved in the study became pregnant. Among the women who had taken only trace element supplements, six experienced NTD pregnancies. There were no cases of NTD births among the women who had taken folic acid along with other nutrients. In analyzing other birth defects, the researchers found similar results: Among the children born to women in the trace element group, forty-one babies were born with congenital malformations, compared with twenty-eight babies born with congenital malformations in the folic acid group.

Cardiovascular Disease

As discussed earlier, scientific evidence now points to folic acid—in addition to vitamins B_6 and B_{12}—as a possible defense against cardiovascular disease. In 1995, researchers from the University of Washington published the results of a survey in which they had evaluated data from twenty-seven separate studies linking high homocysteine levels to cardiovascular disease, and an additional eleven studies of folic acid's effects on homocysteine levels. The results, published in *JAMA (The Journal of the American Medical Association)*, revealed that high homocysteine levels are, indeed, a risk factor for cardiovascular disease.

In a separate study, Canadian scientists reported finding an association between the level of folic acid in the bloodstream and the risk of death from coronary heart disease (CHD). This study involved more than 5,000 men and women, none of whom had showed signs of CHD. At the start of the study in the early 1970s, the researchers measured the participants' blood folic acid levels. Over the next fifteen years, 165 participants died of coronary heart disease. The results of the study, published in 1996, showed that the individuals with the lowest folic acid levels had a 69 percent greater chance of dying from coronary disease than individuals with the highest folic acid levels.

In a 1997 study, researchers in Ireland compared homocysteine levels in 750 men and women with heart disease with homocysteine levels in 800 healthy men and women. Not surprisingly, higher blood levels of homocysteine were strongly associated with a greater risk of heart disease. The researchers discovered that participants who were taking supplements containing folic acid, vitamin B_6, or vitamin B_{12} were 62 percent less likely to have heart disease than those who did not take these supplements—an effect that was due, at least in part, to the lower blood levels of homocysteine in the individuals taking vitamin supplements.

Researchers at Tufts University published a study in *The New England Journal of Medicine* in 1995, reporting that high blood levels of homocysteine are associated with an increased likelihood of severe narrowing of the arteries in the neck, a condition that increases the risk of stroke. Out of more than 1,000 elderly men and women involved in the study, the participants with the highest homocysteine concentrations were twice as likely to have severe narrowing of the arteries, when compared with participants with the lowest homocysteine levels. The researchers also found that individuals with lower blood levels of folic acid and vitamin B_6, as well as lower folic acid intakes, were more likely to have severe narrowing of the arteries.

Cervical Dysplasia

Some research has suggested that folic acid deficiency may cause cervical dysplasia, an abnormal growth of cervical tissues that is considered precancerous. The condition may be caused by the human papillomavirus (HPV), the same virus that causes genital warts, which may be transmitted during sexual intercourse. Fortunately, supplementation with folic acid may protect against cervical dysplasia in women with low blood levels of the vitamin.

In 1992, researchers at the University of Alabama, Birmingham, measured blood levels of several different vitamins and minerals—including folic acid—in 294 women with cervical dysplasia and in 170 women who did not have the condition. The scientists found that women with low levels of folic acid were at greater risk of cervical cancer from factors such as cigarette smoking and HPV infection. Furthermore, women with HPV and low blood levels of folic acid were five times more likely to have cervical dysplasia than women with the virus who had high blood levels of folic acid.

DEFICIENCY SYMPTOMS

Folic acid deficiency causes the appearance of a range of symptoms, including digestive disturbances, sore tongue, fatigue, pallor, memory problems, and paranoia. Deficiency commonly results in a form of anemia characterized by malformed, oversized red blood cells. The signs of this type of anemia include headaches, weakness, heart palpitations, and irritability.

Because the blood symptoms of folic acid deficiency are similar to those associated with vitamin B_{12} deficiency, it is sometimes difficult to determine which nutrient is lacking. Giving extra folate to a person with a B_{12} deficiency may make the blood cells appear normal, leading the health-care practitioner to believe the deficiency has been treated when, in fact, the treatment is simply masking an underlying B_{12} deficiency. And, as we discussed in Chapter 14, vitamin B_{12} deficiency can have serious consequences. By the same token, a folic acid deficiency that is mistakenly treated with extra vitamin B_{12} will cause the deficiency to worsen.

TOXICITY SYMPTOMS

There is no evidence that folic acid causes side effects, even when taken in very large doses. However, high doses of the vitamin may interfere with the body's absorption of zinc. In addition, taking folic acid supplements can mask the signs of a vitamin B_{12} deficiency. Left untreated, pernicious anemia—a blood disorder related to B_{12} deficiency—can lead to serious, permanent nerve damage and paralysis. Finally, high doses of folic acid can also block the action of anticonvulsant medications, so that these drugs are not as effective in preventing seizures. If you have epilepsy and you are considering taking folic acid supplements, be sure to consult with your doctor.

Are You at Risk of Folic Acid Deficiency?

How do you know if you're at risk of folic acid deficiency? Take a moment to review the questions below. If you answer yes to any of these questions, you have an above-average risk of developing a deficiency.

❏ *Have you been diagnosed with vitamin B_{12} deficiency?* Vitamin B_{12} helps the body to use folic acid effectively. Without vitamin B_{12}, folic acid is unable to do its blood-building work, to metabolize amino acids, or to synthesize proteins and nucleic acids.

❏ *Do you have cancer?* Because cancer cells replicate quickly, they use up a lot of folic acid, which can lead to a deficiency.

❏ *Do you take any of the following medications: trimethoprim or anticonvulsant drugs?* Medications that may decrease folic acid levels in the body include trimethoprim, which is used to treat urinary tract infections; and anticonvulsant drugs, such as phenytoin, phenobarbital, and primidone.

❏ *Do you use oral contraceptives?* Birth control pills can decrease folic acid levels in the body.

OPTIMAL DAILY ALLOWANCE

Determining an exact ODA for folic acid is difficult because individual needs for this B vitamin vary according to a range of factors. For this reason, all men and women—no matter what age—should aim to take in 400 to 600 micrograms of the vitamin every day. This range can help prevent cervical dysplasia in older women and will help to reduce the risk of cardiovascular disease in both sexes.

Women of childbearing age should be especially careful to maximize their folic acid intake to prevent neural tube defects and other birth defects.

Food Sources

Folic acid is found in a variety of leafy green vegetables, including spinach, kale, and beet greens; liver and other organ meats; nuts

❏ *Do you drink large amounts of alcohol?* Alcohol decreases the absorption of folic acid. Also, alcoholics tend to substitute alcohol—which has no real nutritional value—for nutrient-dense foods, so they generally don't take in adequate amounts of folic acid and other nutrients.

❏ *Are you pregnant or breast-feeding?* Pregnancy is a time of increased nutritional needs, because the growth of a new person requires every known nutrient. Folic acid is very important in pregnancy to promote normal cell division and cell growth of the fetus, and the expectant mother's own folic acid resources are drawn upon during this time to provide for the developing baby's needs. Breast-feeding mothers are also at increased risk of deficiency because some amount of folic acid is lost in breast milk. Therefore, recent RDA guidelines for women in the first six months of nursing call for an additional 100 micrograms of folic acid per day; thereafter, women who breast-feed should take an extra 80 micrograms of folic acid daily.

❏ *Are you an older person?* Many older people have poor dietary habits, usually because they are on limited budgets or because they live alone and do not cook much for themselves.

and legumes; and asparagus, broccoli, and whole wheat. Also, some ready-to-eat cereals are fortified with the vitamin.

Be aware that cooking and other types of food processing can reduce the folic acid content of foods, and some amount of folic acid may leach into cooking water. In fact, 50 percent or more of the folic acid contained in many foods may be lost due to food processing. Folic acid can also be destroyed by exposure to bright light.

Are You Maximizing Your Folic Acid Intake?

You can reach 400 micrograms of folic acid simply by consuming two glasses of orange juice, one Florida avocado, one cup of boiled lima beans, and one serving of instant oatmeal—or by eating some generous portions of enriched cereals. The average person falls short of the optimal recommendation, however. Government studies show that the average consumption of folic acid in the United States is only 259 micrograms of folic acid per day. If there is any question about the inadequacy of your diet with respect to this nutrient, you should take a folic acid supplement. This issue is so critical for preventing birth defects that the U.S. Public Health Service now recommends that all women of childbearing age should supplement their diets with 400 micrograms of folic acid per day.

You can use the information in Table 16.1 to determine your average daily intake of folic acid. The foods and beverages included in this table are arranged according to the percentage of the Optimal Daily Allowance of folic acid they contain. Remember, the ODA of folic acid ranges from 400 to 600 micrograms. For this self-test, we'll use the lowest ODA in the range, 400 micrograms.

Start by keeping a food diary for at least three to four days; the longer you keep the diary, the more accurate your calculations will be. Write down everything you eat and drink, as well as the estimated serving size, and refer to the table on page 159 to determine the percentage of the ODA that each food or beverage provides. At the end of each day, add up all of the percentages to see if you've reached 100 percent for the day. (If your optimal dose falls elsewhere in the recommended range, take that into account when calculating percentages.)

If you find that, on average, you do not take in 100 percent of your ODA for folic acid, then you may decide that you want to

Table 16.1. Percent of Folic Acid ODA in Common Foods and Beverages

Food	Serving Size	Food	Serving Size
5 Percent		**20 Percent**	
Banana	1 medium	Asparagus, boiled	6 spears
Butternut squash, boiled	$^1/_2$ cup	Avocado, Florida	$^1/_2$ medium
		Bran Flakes cereal	1 ounce
Cashews	1 ounce	Corn Flakes cereal	1 ounce
Cauliflower, boiled	$^1/_2$ cup	Orange juice from concentrate	8 ounces
Corn, yellow, boiled	$^1/_2$ cup		
Cottage cheese, low-fat	1 cup	Raisin Bran cereal	1 ounce
		Turnip greens, boiled	$^1/_2$ cup
Egg	1 large	**30 Percent**	
Endive	$^1/_2$ cup	Lima beans, boiled	1 cup
Grapefruit juice, canned	1 cup	Oatmeal, instant	1 packet
		Spinach, boiled	$^1/_2$ cup
Green beans, boiled	$^1/_2$ cup	**40 Percent**	
Hazelnuts	1 ounce	Broad beans, boiled	1 cup
Okra, boiled	$^1/_2$ cup	Great Northern beans, boiled	1 cup
Peanuts	1 ounce		
Potato, baked, with skin	1 medium	**50 Percent**	
Sweet potato, baked	1 medium	Beef liver, braised	$3^1/_2$ ounces
Tomato juice, canned	6 ounces	Kidney beans, boiled	1 cup
Yogurt, low-fat	8 ounces	**60 Percent**	
10 Percent		Black beans, boiled	1 cup
Artichoke, boiled	1 medium	Navy beans, boiled	1 cup
Avocado, California	$^1/_2$ medium	**70 Percent**	
Beets, boiled	$^1/_2$ cup	Garbanzo beans, boiled	1 cup
Broccoli, boiled	$^1/_2$ cup	**80 Percent**	
Brussels sprouts, boiled	4 sprouts	Black-eyed peas, boiled	1 cup
		Lentils, boiled	1 cup
Orange	1 medium	**100 Percent or More**	
Parsnips	$^1/_2$ cup	Chicken liver, simmered	$3^1/_2$ ounces
Peas, green, boiled	$^1/_2$ cup	Product 19 cereal	1 ounce
Pineapple juice, canned	1 cup	Total cereal	1 ounce

take vitamin supplements for optimal health. But how much of this nutrient do you need to take to reach your ODA? Here's an example of how to perform this calculation: Let's say you determine that you are getting 50 percent (0.50) of your target intake through diet alone. Multiply 0.50 and 400 milligrams (the ODA of folic acid) and you'll find that you're taking in 200 micrograms of folic acid in your diet. To make up the difference, then, you should take 200 micrograms of folic acid daily in supplement form.

Folic acid is most commonly available in 400-microgram tablets. Even if you need to supplement with only 200 micrograms, taking 400 micrograms is fine—you'll easily be able to meet your need without putting your health at risk.

RECOMMENDATIONS

When it comes to nutrition, there's a lot of important information to remember—so it helps to have what you need to know right at your fingertips. The most critical facts about folic acid are summarized below.

What is the Optimal Daily Allowance of folic acid?
The ODA of folic acid for men and women ranges from 400 to 600 micrograms. Women of childbearing age must be especially careful to take in optimal doses of this vitamin.

What circumstances might affect the amount of folic acid you need to take in each day?
Some lifestyle or health factors can affect the amount of folic acid you consume or decrease the amount that your body is able to absorb and use. You'll have to be particularly conscientious about taking in the ODA of folic acid if:

- You have a vitamin B_{12} deficiency.

- You have cancer.

- You take certain medications, including trimethoprim, anticonvulsant drugs, and oral contraceptives.

- You drink large amounts of alcohol.

- You are pregnant or breast-feeding.

- You are an older person.

Is it possible to consume the optimal amount of folic acid through diet alone?

While it is possible to take in the Optimal Daily Allowance of folic acid through dietary sources alone, research shows that many Americans do not reach this intake level. The average folic acid intake in the United States is only 259 micrograms per day—clearly below the ODA range for this vitamin. Considering the facts, then, it seems that many people may very well benefit by taking supplements.

Chapter 17

Vitamin C
(Ascorbic Acid)

No other vitamin has been the subject of as much scientific scrutiny and media attention as vitamin C has been over the years. Certainly, no single nutrient has been claimed to prevent or cure as many diseases and disorders as this vitamin. Thanks in part to vitamin C's most prominent and outspoken advocate, Linus Pauling, millions of people regularly take large amounts of this nutrient in hopes that it might cure them of everything from the common cold to cancer. While experts still disagree about the extent of vitamin C's protective benefits, we do have convincing evidence that the nutrient plays several important health-promoting roles.

FUNCTIONS IN THE BODY

Vitamin C is involved in the formation and maintenance of collagen, a protein that is the chief component of the body's connective tissues, including cartilage, bone, teeth, skin, ligaments, and tendons. Collagen is also part of the supporting material of tiny blood vessels called capillaries, and it forms the scar tissue that heals wounds.

Although the extent of vitamin C's effects on immunity is still in debate, the nutrient is known to play a critical role in many aspects of the body's immune system function. Vitamin C stimulates the production of certain classes of antibodies, which fight invading viruses, bacteria, and fungi to protect the body against ill-

The History of Vitamin C

The story of vitamin C is closely intertwined with the history of the deficiency disease scurvy, a potentially fatal condition that dates back to ancient times. During the height of the Roman Empire, soldiers involved in a two-year campaign along the Rhine River began experiencing sore, bleeding gums and loose teeth—symptoms that would later be identified as classic signs of scurvy. However, these symptoms disappeared when the Roman soldiers consumed a local plant, now believed to have been sorrel, which is rich in vitamin C.

Centuries later, the symptoms of scurvy resurfaced, this time in sailors on long voyages. As far back as the sixteenth century, seafaring men suffered from symptoms that started as weakness and fatigue, followed by inflamed, bleeding gums and loose teeth, as well as bruising. In a journal entry in 1593, Sir Richard Hawkins described the deaths of 10,000 sailors from severe deficiencies associated with scurvy. In his desperate search for a treatment for this disease, Hawkins discovered that the condition was reversed when his men ate oranges and lemons. As effective as this treatment was, however, it fell out of favor for unknown reasons, and scurvy reemerged on a large scale, claiming many more lives over the next century.

Finally, in the mid-1700s, a physician and surgeon of the British fleet named James Lind revived Hawkins' antidote for scurvy. Dr. Lind noticed that the incidence of scurvy was lower among the men on ships with food supplies that included citrus fruits, which were used primarily to flavor the large amounts of fish in the diet. Through experimentation, Dr. Lind clearly showed that scurvy-stricken sailors who ate two oranges and one lemon each day were ready to return to duty in about a week. He advised that lemon juice be added to the sailors' diets. In 1804, the British Navy ordered lime juice rations for its sailors. The result was a dramatic drop in the incidence of scurvy among British sailors. It has never completely disappeared, however; the condition is still present in emerging countries where nutritional deficiencies are commonplace.

It wasn't until 1932—almost 200 years after Dr. Lind's discovery—that Hungarian scientist Albert Szent-Gyorgyi isolated and identified vitamin C as the specific nutrient in fruits and vegetables responsible for preventing scurvy. Appropriately, the vitamin was called *ascorbic acid,* which literally means "no scurvy."

nesses and infections. It also promotes the production of *interferon*, a protein that protects cells from viral infection.

Of course, vitamin C is also known as an antioxidant that appears to help protect the body against some of the potentially damaging chemical reactions of oxygen. In particular, it interferes with the production and activity of free radicals, the unstable molecules that steal electrons from healthy cells in the body. Experts believe that oxidative damage is connected to the development of many degenerative diseases, such as cancer and cardiovascular disease, and may accelerate the aging process.

Additionally, vitamin C blocks the formation of *nitrosamines*, potentially cancer-causing compounds that are produced in the stomach from nitrites—antimicrobial agents found in foods such as ham, sausages, and hot dogs. Nitrosamines have been associated with an increased risk of certain cancers, especially those of the digestive system.

Another valuable function of vitamin C is that it enhances the absorption of iron from the intestinal tract. It appears to do this by binding with the iron and "smuggling" it through the intestinal lining, so that a greater percentage of the iron that's consumed is actually absorbed. The vitamin can also increase or decrease the absorption of other minerals. For example, vitamin C may slightly decrease the body's absorption of copper. This function is particularly important for people affected by Wilson's disease, a disorder in which the body cannot properly metabolize copper. The result of this disease is a toxic accumulation of the trace element that can damage the brain, kidneys, and liver. By binding with copper and helping to carry the excess out of the body, vitamin C can reduce copper levels and lessen the effects of Wilson's disease. Finally, vitamin C has also been shown to stimulate the elimination of lead in body tissues. Among other effects, high blood levels of lead can cause impaired intelligence in children.

In high doses, vitamin C can minimize allergic reactions by interfering with the release of a chemical called *histamine*. The immune system releases histamine when it reacts to an allergen, a substance that provokes an allergic response. Histamine causes the symptoms commonly associated with allergies, including frequent sneezing, itchy or watery eyes, and runny nose.

HEALTH BENEFITS

Over the years, you've probably heard the claims that vitamin C has a very powerful ability to fight both mild and serious diseases. A considerable body of research has been compiled on vitamin C, and some of the scientific evidence is persuasive and promising.

Inevitably, some of the claims for vitamin C have not panned out—at least not to the extent that its proponents would have you believe. But research does show that the vitamin promotes wound healing, helps keep gums healthy, and even reduces the risk of iron-deficiency anemia. Vitamin C may also protect against development of cataracts, cardiovascular disease, and some forms of cancer.

The Common Cold

Despite the claims of respected scientists such as the late Linus Pauling, no definitive evidence exists that large doses of vitamin C can prevent or cure the common cold. Beginning back in the 1970s, three carefully conducted studies that took place in Canada examined the role of vitamin C in fighting colds. The researchers could not confirm that the nutrient reduced the number of colds, although there was some indication that vitamin C can help individuals recover more quickly from upper respiratory infections. Taken in large doses, the vitamin also appears to provide modest symptomatic relief, probably due to its antihistamine action.

Cancer

One doesn't have to look far to find evidence supporting vitamin C's role as a cancer-preventing agent—a number of large-scale studies have linked a higher vitamin C intake with a reduced risk of cancer. But what gives the nutrient its powerful punch?

Researchers have found that vitamin C possesses a variety of anticancer properties. First, there is its status as an antioxidant that can neutralize damaging free radicals before they can harm healthy cells. Then there's vitamin C's role as an immune system enhancer. And finally, the nutrient is an important factor in preventing the formation of cancer-causing nitrosamines in the stomach.

Breast Cancer

In a 1990 study, investigators at the University of Toronto and other major medical centers collected and analyzed the data gathered from a number of existing studies of vitamin C's effects on breast cancer in women. The researchers found that a high vitamin C intake provided substantial protection against breast cancer. As a matter of fact, women who consumed the most vitamin C were 31 percent less likely to develop breast cancer than women who consumed the least amounts of the vitamin.

Cervical Cancer

Researchers at the Fred Hutchinson Cancer Research Center and the University of Washington, Seattle, calculated vitamin C intake, as well as the intake of vitamins A and E and folic acid, based on questionnaire responses of over 400 women. Of the participants, 189 women had been diagnosed with cervical cancer, while 227 women were cancer-free. The results of the study, published in 1989, indicated that high vitamin C intakes reduced the risk of developing cervical cancer. Women who ranked in the highest 25 percent for vitamin C consumption were only half as likely to develop cervical cancer as women in the lowest 25 percent.

Lung Cancer

Over a period of twenty years, researchers in Finland monitored the health of more than 4,500 men to determine how their antioxidant intake influenced their risk of developing lung cancer. During the course of the study, 117 cases of lung cancer were diagnosed. Among nonsmoking participants in the study, those who took in the lowest levels of vitamin C were three times more likely to develop lung cancer than those who consumed the highest levels of the nutrient.

Starting in the early 1970s, researchers at the National Cancer Institute took the dietary histories of more than 4,500 men and women to determine their intake levels of various nutrients. Then, over the next two decades, the researchers monitored the health of the participants. The results of the study, published in 1997, revealed that higher intakes of dietary vitamin C are indeed associated with a lower risk of lung cancer. Among the participants, individuals who consumed the greatest amounts of vitamin C were 34 percent less likely to develop lung cancer than those who took in the least amounts.

Oral Cancer

A 1988 study conducted jointly at several research centers in the United States examined the effects of vitamin C intake on 871 men and women with oral cancer and 979 cancer-free individuals. The researchers found that individuals who consumed the most vitamin C had a 40 to 50 percent lower risk of developing oral cancer than participants who consumed the least.

In another study, cancer researchers in northern California analyzed the dietary intakes of 141 men and women with cancer of the salivary glands, and then compared the results with those of similarly aged men and women who did not have cancer. The most notable discovery was that individuals who consumed more than 200 milligrams of vitamin C daily were 60 percent less likely to develop cancer of the salivary glands than people who consumed 100 milligrams or less.

Other Forms of Cancer

Gladys Block, a researcher at the School of Public Health of the University of California, Berkeley, recently evaluated the abundance of scientific literature now available about vitamin C's protective effects against cancer. The results of her evaluation are as follows:

- All studies that have looked at the link between vitamin C and rectal cancer have concluded that higher intakes of the vitamin reduced the risk of this form of cancer.

- Nine of ten studies have found about a two-fold decrease in the likelihood of developing cancer of the esophagus when vitamin C intake increased.

- Eight of nine studies concluded that increasing vitamin C intake decreases the risk of developing stomach cancer.

Positive results were also cited relative to vitamin C and the prevention of cancers of the cervix, colon, lungs, and pancreas.

Vitamin C intake did not seem to significantly affect the development of ovarian or prostate cancer, however.

Cardiovascular Disease

Some studies have shown that vitamin C may lower total cholesterol, reduce "bad" low-density lipoprotein (LDL) cholesterol, and increase "good" high-density lipoprotein (HDL) cholesterol. A daily intake of 1 to 2 grams of vitamin C has been shown to increase HDL cholesterol levels.

Using data from the First National Health and Nutrition Examination Survey (NHANES I) conducted by the National Center for Health Statistics between 1971 and 1975, scientists examined the relationship between vitamin C consumption and deaths caused by cardiovascular disease. Mortality attributed to cardiovascular disease was 42 percent lower in men with the highest vitamin C intakes than in men with the lowest intakes. In women, the difference was 25 percent. High intake of vitamin C reduced the number of deaths from any causes (including cardiovascular disease) by 35 percent in men and 10 percent in women.

In a 1984 study published by researchers in Japan, 194 men were divided into three groups based on their intake of vitamin C. The average systolic blood pressure reading of the men who consumed the most vitamin C was 7 percent lower than the average systolic reading of the men who consumed the least; the average diastolic reading was 6 percent lower. Hypertension was seven times more common in the group with the lowest intakes of vitamin C, compared with the group that had the highest intakes.

Research conducted in Finland in 1988 looked at the correlation between blood levels of vitamin C and blood pressure. The study involved 722 men who were divided into four groups according to their blood levels of vitamin C. Results showed that the average systolic and diastolic blood pressure readings of the group with the highest blood levels of vitamin C were about 5 percent below the average of the group with the lowest levels of the nutrient.

Cataracts

The aqueous fluid within the eye, which fills the space between the cornea and the lens, normally contains a high amount of vitamin C. With increasing age, however, vitamin C levels in this front part of the eye begin to decline. As levels of the antioxidant decrease, proteins in the lens of the eye become more susceptible to oxidation. The resulting damage to the lens causes a cataract—a clouding of the lens within the eye. Fortunately, adequate vitamin C intake may protect against cataracts, or at least delay their onset.

A study conducted in 1991 at Brigham and Women's Hospital, Boston, looked at the effects of vitamin C consumption on 77 men and women with cataracts and on 35 cataract-free individuals. The results showed that low vitamin C intake is associated with an increased risk of developing cataracts. Individuals in the bottom 20 percent for vitamin C intake were four times more likely to develop cataracts than those in the top 20 percent.

In 1997, researchers at Tufts University investigated the effect of vitamin C supplements on the development of lens opacities—a precursor to cataracts—in 247 middle-aged and elderly women. The researchers found that women who had taken vitamin C supplements for more than ten years had a 77 percent lower risk of developing early lens opacity than those not taking supplements.

Longevity

In a study published in 1992 by researchers at the University of California, Los Angeles, investigators examined dietary habits—including intake of vitamin C from both food and supplement sources—of more than 11,000 men and women, and then monitored the health of the participants over the course of ten years. The researchers concluded that men who consumed the most vitamin C (about 150 milligrams daily) had a 35 percent lower death rate during the ten years than men who consumed the least vitamin C (about 30 milligrams daily). Women who took in the highest amounts of vitamin C had a 10 percent lower death rate than women who took in the least amounts. Data analysis showed that high vitamin C intake increased the life expectancy of men by six years and of women by one year.

Memory

Some scientists think that memory loss associated with aging may be, at least in part, a result of damage to brain cells—damage that could be prevented with antioxidants such as vitamin C. According to this theory, increased consumption of antioxidants could potentially slow or prevent memory loss as we age.

Swiss researchers published a study in 1997 that revealed a possible association between vitamin C and memory performance. Blood samples were taken from 442 men and women between sixty-five and ninety-four years old, and blood levels of various antioxidant vitamins—including vitamin C—were measured. The participants in the study were also tested for memory function. As it turned out, men and women with higher blood levels of vitamin C performed significantly better on almost all tests of memory than participants with lower levels of the nutrient.

DEFICIENCY SYMPTOMS

Because vitamin C is water-soluble, it is not stored in the body, but is quickly excreted. Thus, the nutrient must be replenished regularly. Fortunately, maintaining an adequate intake of vitamin C is relatively easy, since the vitamin is plentiful in a wide variety of fruits and vegetables. This is why serious deficiencies are rare in developed countries. Even mild vitamin C deficiencies are relatively rare; these are usually associated with some illness or lifestyle habit that interferes with the body's intake or utilization of vitamin C. For example, smoking, stress, diabetes, and chronic diseases can increase the body's need for vitamin C. A mild deficiency may produce symptoms such as fatigue, loss of appetite, muscle weakness, and greater susceptibility to infections.

The classic deficiency disease associated with vitamin C is *scurvy,* a name that comes from the Italian *scorbutico,* referring to a discontented, neurotic person. The condition is seldom seen in the United States, and usually occurs only in some bottle-fed infants, in elderly people, and in alcoholics. Most of the symptoms of scurvy develop because of the breakdown of collagen that occurs in the absence of vitamin C. These include: rough, dry, scaly skin; swollen, bleeding gums and loose teeth; hemorrhaging in blood vessels; slow healing of wounds; bone and joint pain; and an increased susceptibility to infections. Anemia is also a common symptom of severe vitamin C deficiency, because vitamin C helps

Are You at Risk of Vitamin C Deficiency?

How do you know if you're at risk of vitamin C deficiency? Take a moment to review the questions below. If you answer yes to any of these questions, you have an above-average risk of developing a deficiency.

❑ *Do you have diabetes?* Studies show that people with diabetes have lower blood levels of vitamin C than people who do not have the disease. This is because ascorbic acid enters cells via the same protein carrier as glucose, or blood sugar. When glucose levels are high, as they are in individuals with diabetes, glucose rather than ascorbic acid is absorbed into the body cells; since the ascorbic acid is not used by the body, more is excreted in the urine.

❑ *Do you take either of the following medications: aspirin or tetracycline?* Aspirin interferes with vitamin C absorption; the antibiotic tetracycline increases the rate at which vitamin C is broken down in the body.

❑ *Do you use oral contraceptives?* Birth control pills increase excretion of the vitamin in the urine.

❑ *Are you under any sort of physical or mental stress?* Vitamin C is an important factor in our ability to handle all types of stresses. The body's normal levels of ascorbic acid are especially depleted during high-stress occurrences, such as surgery, or any kind of illness, including infections and injuries.

❑ *Are you exposed to environmental pollutants?* Exposure to environmental pollutants increases the body's need for vitamin C, because the nutrient must work overtime as an antioxidant to detoxify the body. Vitamin C is also necessary for the proper func-

the body to absorb and use iron. Other warning signs of scurvy are lethargy, fatigue, and change in personality.

TOXICITY SYMPTOMS

Vitamin C is reported to be relatively safe for most people, even when consumed in large quantities over long periods of time. Doses as high as 10 grams per day—more than 100 times the

tion of several enzyme systems that help detoxify pollutants, as well as harmful drugs, minimizing their effects on the body.

❏ *Do you drink large amounts of alcohol?* Some researchers believe that alcohol destroys vitamin C, while others believe that another, still undefined mechanism may be at work. Also, alcoholics tend to substitute alcohol—which has no real nutritional value—for nutrient-dense foods, so they generally don't take in adequate amounts of vitamin C and other nutrients.

❏ *Do you smoke cigarettes?* Studies show that the need for vit amin C is twice as high in smokers as in nonsmokers, because smoking increases the rate at which vitamin C is broken down in the body. Additionally, cigarette smoke causes oxidative damage to the body's healthy cells and tissues. People who smoke need greater amounts of antioxidants such as vitamin C to neutralize free radicals.

❏ *Are you on a "fad" diet?* Many weight-loss programs include foods that are low in vitamin C.

❏ *Are you pregnant or breast-feeding?* Pregnancy is a time of increased nutritional needs because the growth of a new person requires every known nutrient. Women who are breast-feeding need to take in adequate vitamin C to compensate for the 18 to 22 milligrams lost in breast milk.

❏ *Are you an older person?* Older people often take medications that accelerate vitamin C breakdown. This is compounded by the fact that many older people have poor dietary habits, often because they are on limited budgets or because they live alone and do not cook much for themselves.

RDA—taken for several years are safe for many people because any vitamin C the body can't use is excreted in the urine, thus preventing toxic buildup. Be aware, however, that this is not the case for everyone who decides to supplement with vitamin C. Some studies have shown that adverse symptoms can occur with daily doses of as little as 1 gram.

The most common symptom that results from excessive vitamin C intake is intestinal gas and diarrhea, often accompanied by nausea and headache. To avoid experiencing the discomforts associated with excessive intake of vitamin C, try increasing your vitamin C intake gradually by adding an extra 100 milligrams per week to your daily dose.

You may have heard that large doses of vitamin C increase the risk of developing kidney stones. This is a rare problem that probably occurs only at extremely high doses, and then only in people who are already highly susceptible to kidney stone formation. But you should know that vitamin C may interfere with certain diagnostic tests used by physicians. For example, large amounts of vitamin C in the urine may produce inaccurate results on the urine glucose test used to screen for diabetes. The nutrient can also cause a false negative result for the fecal occult blood test that is used to diagnose colon cancer.

Doctors have also reported a condition they call "rebound scurvy" that may occur in people who suddenly stop taking vitamin C after having supplemented with large doses of the nutrient. The body continues to rapidly break down and clear out vitamin C as though large levels of the nutrient were still being consumed, causing some of the milder symptoms of scurvy, such as bleeding gums. This effect can easily be avoided by decreasing vitamin C intake gradually, rather than stopping supplementation abruptly.

OPTIMAL DAILY ALLOWANCE

Although the RDA of vitamin C for men and women is 60 milligrams, you may benefit from higher doses—possibly even ten times higher. With all of the positive evidence that has accumulated about vitamin C's protective effects against cardiovascular disease, some forms of cancer, and cataracts, the case for increasing vitamin C intake has become more persuasive. For this reason, the ODA of vitamin C ranges from 250 to 500 milligrams. The higher levels are appropriate for people who are at an above-average risk of deficiency.

Food Sources

Many plant and animal foods contain moderate or high amounts of vitamin C. Especially good sources of the nutrient include broccoli, Brussels sprouts, collards, kale, turnip greens, parsley, sweet peppers, strawberries, cabbage, cauliflower, mustard greens, and spinach. Sources of moderate amounts of vitamin C are potatoes, some citrus fruits (grapefruit, limes, tangerines), lima beans, melons, turnips, beef, poultry, fish, and dairy products. Grains do not contain vitamin C.

Vitamin C is easily destroyed when it is exposed to heat and light, and it is highly unstable in the presence of water. The methods used to prepare foods can affect their vitamin C content, as well—even chopping food into smaller sections can cause a rapid decline in a food's supply of the nutrient.

Are You Maximizing Your Vitamin C Intake?

While statistics show that most American men and women take in more than the RDA of vitamin C, it seems that a great many people fail to reach the recommended ODA range for this vitamin. For those people who do not take in optimal amounts of vitamin C from dietary sources alone, it's pretty likely that supplementation will be beneficial. Where do you stand?

You can use the information in Table 17.1 to determine your average daily intake of vitamin C. The foods and beverages included in this table are arranged according to the percentage of the Optimal Daily Allowance of vitamin C they contain. Remember, the ODA of vitamin C ranges from 250 to 500 milligrams. For this self-test, we'll use the highest ODA in the range, 500 milligrams.

Start by keeping a food diary for at least three to four days; the longer you keep the diary, the more accurate your calculations will be. Write down everything you eat and drink, as well as the estimated serving size, and refer to the table on page 176 to determine the percentage of the ODA that each food or beverage provides. At the end of each day, add up all of the percentages to see if you've reached 100 percent for the day. (If your optimal dose falls elsewhere in the recommended range, take that into account when calculating percentages.)

If you find that, on average, you do not take in 100 percent of your ODA for vitamin C, then you may decide that you want to take vitamin supplements for optimal health. But how much of this nutrient do you need to take to reach your ODA? Here's an

Table 17.1. Percent of Vitamin C ODA in Common Foods and Beverages

Food	Serving Size	Food	Serving Size
5 Percent		Tomato juice, canned	6 ounces
Acorn squash, baked	1 cup	**10 Percent**	
Brussels sprouts	4 sprouts	Broccoli, boiled	½ cup
Butternut squash, baked	1 cup	Grapefruit juice, canned	1 cup
Cantaloupe pieces	½ cup	Kiwi fruit	1 medium
Cauliflower	½ cup	Mango	1 medium
Grapefruit	½ medium	Orange	1 medium
Honeydew melon pieces	½ cup	Papaya	½ medium
Kale, boiled	½ cup	Pepper, sweet	½ cup
Lemon	1 medium	Product 19 cereal	1 cup
Marinara sauce	1 cup	**20 Percent**	
Peas, green, boiled	½ cup	Cranberry juice cocktail	1 cup
Pineapple juice, canned	1 cup	Orange juice from concentrate	1 cup
Potato, baked, with skin	1 medium	**30 Percent**	
Strawberries	½ cup	Guava	1 medium
Sweet potato, baked	1 medium	**100 Percent or More**	
		Acerola	½ cup

example of how to perform this calculation: Let's say you determine that you are getting 30 percent (0.30) of your vitamin C target through diet alone. Multiply 0.30 and 500 milligrams (the ODA of vitamin C) and you'll find that you are consuming 150 milligrams of vitamin C in your diet. To make up the difference, then, you should take in 350 milligrams of vitamin C in supplement form.

Because vitamin C is commonly sold in doses of 250 and 500 milligrams, you may have difficulty getting supplements of the precise amount you want. Try to come as close to your target intake as possible without taking several tablets to make things come out even. If you need a 350-milligram supplement, you can go a little higher and take a 500-milligram tablet, which is more than adequate to meet your needs without any health risks.

RECOMMENDATIONS

When it comes to nutrition, there's a lot of important information to remember—so it helps to have what you need to know right at your fingertips. The most critical facts about vitamin C are summarized below.

What is the Optimal Daily Allowance of vitamin C?
The ODA of vitamin C for men and women ranges from 250 to 500 milligrams. It's best to aim for the higher end of this suggested intake range.

What circumstances might affect the amount of vitamin C you need to take in each day?
Some lifestyle or health factors can affect the amount of vitamin C you consume or decrease the amount that your body is able to absorb and use. You'll have to be particularly conscientious about taking in the ODA of vitamin C if:

- You have diabetes.

- You take certain medications, including aspirin and tetracycline.

- You use oral contraceptives.

- You are under any sort of physical or mental stress.

- You are exposed to environmental pollutants.

- You drink large amounts of alcohol.

- You are on a "fad" diet.

- You are pregnant or breast-feeding.

- You are an older person.

Is it possible to consume the optimal amount of vitamin C through diet alone?
Generally speaking, American men and women do consume much more than the RDA of vitamin C. However, according to statistics, the average individual does not take in enough vitamin C from dietary sources to reach the ODA range of the vitamin. Therefore, it seems that many people would benefit from supplementation.

Part Three

The Minerals

Chapter 18

Calcium

Calcium, the most abundant mineral in the human body, makes up about 2 percent of your body weight. The mineral is best known for its role in building and maintaining strong bones, since approximately 99 percent of the body's calcium is contained in the skeleton. The remaining 1 percent—about two-thirds of a tablespoon—is found in the blood and fluids that bathe the body's cells. Although only a small percentage of the body's total calcium content, this minute amount is vital to survival because, among other things, it is required for heart muscle contraction and regulation of the heartbeat.

The body has a built-in mechanism designed to keep blood levels of the mineral balanced—sometimes at the expense of the bones. If the concentration of calcium in the blood dips too low, the parathyroid glands secrete a hormone called *parathormone* that draws stored calcium out of the bones. In this way, the skeleton serves as a sort of "bank" from which calcium can be withdrawn for any number of essential functions in the body. On the other hand, *calcitonin* is secreted by the thyroid gland when the blood concentration of calcium rises too high. This causes calcium to be deposited in the bones and slows absorption of the mineral from the intestine.

FUNCTIONS IN THE BODY

Calcium is essential for mineralization, the process by which bone tissue hardens. Calcium phosphate salts, along with small amounts of other minerals—especially magnesium—gradually crystallize on a foundation of the protein collagen, which causes the bone to become strong and solid. But even though it's rigid, bone tissue is living tissue that is continuously broken down and rebuilt, or remodeled, throughout life. Therefore, adequate intake of calcium and bone-building minerals is important at every stage of life to support the ongoing formation of bone.

Of course, calcium is essential to other body processes besides bone formation. It is needed for the normal contraction and relaxation of every muscle in the body, including the heart. It also controls the release of neurotransmitters, the chemical messengers that transmit impulses along nerve cells, or neurons, throughout the body. Additionally, calcium promotes the process of blood clotting by interacting with blood platelets and by stimulating the proteins necessary for clotting. And it activates several enzyme systems that support biochemical reactions throughout the body.

Some studies indicate that calcium may play an important role in blood pressure regulation, and that deficiency may contribute to hypertension (high blood pressure) in some people. The possibility of such a deficiency should be considered in anyone who has high blood pressure, although it is unlikely that calcium deficiency alone could account for severe—or even moderate—cases of hypertension.

HEALTH BENEFITS

Scientists are continuing to study the effects of calcium on osteoporosis, and while it has become clear that this mineral cannot stop or reverse the process of bone loss, evidence indicates that calcium supplementation later in life will slow the rate of bone loss. Meanwhile, additional research has focused on other potential health benefits of calcium, including its role in regulating blood pressure, and the possible effects on colon cancer.

Osteoporosis

As mentioned above, bone tissue is continuously rebuilt throughout life, as the calcium that gives bones their density and strength is removed and replaced. Osteoporosis occurs when calcium withdrawal from bones exceeds its deposit over an extended period of time, causing the bones to become weaker and more susceptible to fractures. As the spinal vertebrae lose calcium, they become subject to compression fractures, and literally begin to collapse on themselves. This causes a loss of height and a hunched-over appearance, or "dowager's hump." Osteoporosis can also cause the jawbone to become too weak to hold teeth firmly in place, resulting in tooth loss.

Osteoporosis is generally thought of as a problem for older women, because it commonly occurs after menopause—about 25 percent of women over the age of sixty are affected by this condition. However, some younger people and older men are also at risk of developing this disorder. In fact, the process that puts many people at risk of osteoporosis typically begins much earlier in life.

Bone mass—the amount of mineral in the bones—normally increases until some time between the ages of twenty-five and forty, when peak bone mass is achieved. At this point, the bones are as strong as they ever will be. After that, bone mass and bone strength begin to decrease. In women, bone loss accelerates rapidly after menopause because of the sharp decline in estrogen levels.

Eating a calcium-rich diet during the first four decades of life is important in preventing osteoporosis, because it builds bones to their maximum potential before bone mass begins to decrease. After the age of forty, adequate calcium intake is still important, but it will have less of an impact on bone mass and strength than it did earlier in life. While high calcium intake later in life will *slow* the rate of bone loss, it will not *stop* the process completely or reverse the damage that has occurred.

Many studies document the importance of adequate calcium intake throughout life for bone health. In 1992, researchers at Indiana University's School of Medicine reported on the effects of calcium supplementation on bone density in forty-five sets of identical twins, ranging in age from six to fourteen years old. Over three years, one member of each pair took a 1,000-milligram supplement of calcium citrate malate daily, while the other took a placebo, with no active ingredients. The researchers measured bone density in both groups at intervals during the course of the study. In the children who had not reached puberty, bone density increased in both supplemented and unsupplemented twins, but the increase was 1.4 percent greater in the group taking the calcium supplements. Perhaps surprisingly, this particular study found no significant differences among the older children.

In 1993, researchers at Pennsylvania State University studied the effects of calcium supplementation on bone density in ninety-four teenaged girls. Over the course of eighteen months, one group of girls took a 500-milligram calcium citrate malate supplement daily, while the rest took a placebo. Measurements taken at the beginning and end of the study indicated that bone density increased more in the girls taking calcium than in the girls taking the placebo. The average increase was an extra 24 grams—1.3 percent of skeletal mass—annually during adolescent growth.

A study conducted at the U.S. Department of Agriculture's Human Nutrition Research Center on Aging at Tufts University in Massachusetts examined the effect of calcium supplementation on bone loss in 301 postmenopausal women. In this study, published in 1990, women were divided into three groups: The first group took 500 milligrams of a calcium carbonate supplement per day; the second group supplemented with 500 milligrams of calcium citrate malate per day; and the third group took a placebo. The researchers found that women who had gone through menopause within the five years prior to the study continued to lose bone rapidly, despite taking more calcium. However, those who had gone through menopause at least six years earlier significantly decreased their bone loss by increasing their calcium intake. Of these participants, the women who were most likely to benefit from calcium supplementation were those who had low dietary intakes of calcium before the study began. While both calcium supplements prevented further losses in the bones of the extremities, only calcium citrate malate supplements stopped bone loss in the spinal vertebrae.

French investigators monitored 3,270 older women for eighteen months to determine how supplementation with both calcium and vitamin D affected the incidence of bone fractures. Half the women took supplements of 1.2 grams of calcium and 800 international units of vitamin D daily; the other half took a placebo. In 1992, the researchers reported that the women who took supplements had 43 percent fewer hip fractures during the course of the study, compared with the women who took the placebo.

Measurements taken at the beginning and end of the study revealed that bone density increased by an average of 2.7 percent in the women who took supplements and decreased an average of 4.6 percent in women in the placebo group.

Hypertension

Calcium plays an important role in maintaining normal cardiovascular function. This seems to be due, in part, to its effect on blood pressure. Recent studies have shown that calcium supplements can reduce blood pressure in some people, at least over the short term.

In one study, which included detailed physical examinations and nutritional assessments of 15,000 adults, researchers found that the people with higher blood calcium levels tended to have lower blood pressure readings. Calcium was one of the few dietary components consistently linked with blood pressure readings.

Another study of calcium's effects on blood pressure involved ninety male participants, ages sixteen to twenty-nine, all with mild hypertension. Half of the men took 1 gram of calcium daily for twelve weeks, while the other half took a placebo. The results showed that diastolic blood pressure dropped in both groups; however, the average decrease was significantly greater in the men who took supplemental calcium (4.5 points compared with 2.1). The decline in blood pressure seen in the placebo group was probably due to the "placebo effect"—that is, the positive response may have occurred because these men believed they were receiving active treatment.

Colon Cancer

Some research has indicated that high calcium intake may be associated with a reduced risk of colon cancer. For example, in a nineteen-year-long multicenter study of 1,954 men, researchers compared the calcium and vitamin D intakes of the men who developed colon cancer with intakes of the men who did not. The participants who were free of this cancer had consumed roughly 10 to 15 percent more of these nutrients than the individuals with cancer.

In another study, reported in 1999, researchers examined the possible benefits of calcium supplementation in patients who had had colorectal adenomas (precancerous lesions). More than 900 men and women, all of whom had one or more adenomas removed in the previous three months, participated in the study. For up to four years, half of the participants took 1,200 milligrams of calcium daily, while the other half took a placebo. At the end of the study, the researchers found that the men and women who took calcium had a lower rate of recurrence of adenomas. The results showed that calcium supplements reduced the risk of a recurrence by 19 percent.

Are You at Risk of Calcium Deficiency?

How do you know if you're at risk of calcium deficiency? Take a moment to review the questions below. If you answer yes to any of these questions, you have an above-average risk of developing a deficiency.

❏ *Are you at risk of vitamin D deficiency, or already deficient in the vitamin?* Vitamin D enhances the absorption of calcium in the intestine, and it regulates the level of calcium in the blood. If your diet is low in vitamin D, or if you don't get enough sunlight, your body may not be able to absorb and/or use calcium efficiently.

❏ *Do you use diuretics?* Some diuretics can alter kidney function, causing more calcium to be excreted in the urine.

❏ *Are you very physically active?* Some calcium is lost through perspiration. Therefore, if you are extremely active physically, or if you exercise or engage in strenuous activities in very hot weather, you are at a greater risk of deficiency.

❏ *Are you on a low-calorie diet?* Many people on diets tend to cut back drastically on their intake of calcium-rich foods, particularly dairy products. This problem can be avoided by switching to low-fat and nonfat dairy products, instead of eliminating them from the diet completely.

❏ *Is your diet high in protein?* Evidence suggests that high-protein diets tend to increase the body's excretion of calcium in the urine.

DEFICIENCY SYMPTOMS

Blood and bone levels of calcium in the body are regulated not only by calcium intake, but also by the interaction of calcitonin and parathormone. If calcium intake is adequate, blood and bone levels of the nutrient fluctuate only slightly. However, if calcium intake is low for an extended period of time, the mineral is continuously drawn from the bones to keep the calcium concentration in the blood and other organs at a safe level. Eventually, the excessive loss of calcium from the bones can result in the development of osteoporosis.

❑ *Is your diet high in fat?* Fats can bind to calcium and interfere with its absorption by the body.

❑ *Is your diet very high in fiber?* Compounds called phytates, which are found primarily in fiber-rich whole grains and beans, bind to calcium and interfere with its absorption.

❑ *Is your diet high in phosphorus?* Foods rich in phosphorus—such as beef, pork, chicken, seafood, cheese, and nuts—can interfere with the body's absorption of calcium.

❑ *Are you pregnant or breast-feeding?* Pregnancy is a time of increased nutritional needs because the growth of a new person requires every known nutrient. At birth, the average infant has about 30 grams of calcium in its body, all of which comes from its mother. A pregnant woman who fails to make up for this "loss" by increasing her own calcium consumption puts herself at risk for calcium deficiency. Women who are breast-feeding should also take in adequate calcium to compensate for the 300 milligrams of the mineral that is contained in each quart of breast milk.

❑ *Are you an older person?* Calcium absorption declines after about age seventy, because vitamin D is not as active in the body. Also, people who are housebound and do not get much natural sunlight are more prone to calcium deficiency because the body cannot manufacture vitamin D. This is compounded by the fact that many older people have poor dietary habits, usually because they are on limited budgets or because they live alone and do not cook much for themselves.

While osteoporosis primarily affects postmenopausal women, it may also develop in older men and individuals who are chronically underweight. People who are not physically active are at greater risk as well, since bone mass increases or decreases in direct proportion to the demand put on it. (Weight-bearing exercises—including jogging, dancing, jumping rope, and lifting weights—have been shown to be the best physical activities for increasing bone mass.) Other risk factors include smoking, which more than doubles a person's risk of developing osteoporosis, and excessive use of alcohol, which appears to suppress the growth of new bone.

Bone loss associated with osteoporosis usually goes unnoticed until significant loss has occurred. Unfortunately, it's very common for a person with this condition to be completely unaware of it until what should have been a minor accident causes a broken bone. The bones become so fragile that the person may suffer a fracture just from lifting a child, bending over, receiving a hug, or even sneezing. Each year, about 1.3 million older people in the United States experience fractures related to osteoporosis. These may occur in any bone in the body, but most fractures affect the hip, spine, and wrist bones.

In children, poor absorption of calcium can contribute to the development of rickets, in which the bones fail to grow properly and become soft and pliable (see Chapter 6). This causes the bones to become misshapen, resulting in skeletal problems such as bowed legs, knock-knees, enlarged ankles and wrists, abnormal curvature of the spine, bulging forehead, and narrowed chest. In adults, calcium deficiency can lead to osteomalacia—frequently called adult rickets—which also causes bones to soften, making them more prone to fractures. Signs of osteomalacia include deformities of the limbs and spine, and rheumatic- or arthritic-like pain.

When calcium deficiency is very severe, the concentration of calcium in the blood may fall low enough to produce symptoms elsewhere in the body. This can include a condition called *tetany*, which causes uncomfortable muscle spasms, and modest increases in blood pressure.

TOXICITY SYMPTOMS

Calcium consumption—even in large doses—is rarely associated with serious adverse effects because the body's normal mechanisms are designed to maintain blood levels of this mineral within a safe range. However, very high consumption of calcium (several grams per day) may cause constipation, particularly in older people. Rarely, excessive calcium intake can overwhelm the mechanisms that maintain calcium balance, resulting in symptoms such as drowsiness, weakness, nausea and vomiting, and mental and emotional disturbances, including depression and irritability. In some cases of chronic calcium overload, individuals may develop calcification of soft tissues, including the kidneys.

One recent study suggests that the development of calcium toxicity may depend on the source of the mineral. In this study, high calcium intake from food sources was associated with a decreased risk of developing kidney stones, while high calcium intake from supplements increased the risk of stones. For this reason, you should try to meet your calcium needs with calcium-rich foods, using supplements only as necessary to reach the level of the ODA.

OPTIMAL DAILY ALLOWANCE

The Optimal Daily Allowance of calcium is 1,500 milligrams. This allowance is appropriate for all adults, including men, since there is some evidence that if men lived as long as women, the incidence of osteoporosis would be similar in both sexes.

Because osteoporosis tends to occur later in life, many people assume they do not need to worry about calcium intake while they are young. Nothing could be further from the truth. There is a narrow window of opportunity for building bones to their maximum potential strength. For most people, peak bone mass is achieved by about the age of thirty-five. Once that happens, the ability to build additional bone strength by natural means is lost.

The more bone you have when you reach your peak bone strength, the more you can lose without developing bone fractures. So, if your bones are strong at the age of thirty-five, your risk of osteoporosis is greatly reduced. If they are weak, osteoporosis is almost inevitable. Extra calcium consumption after that point will help protect your bones against further loss, but it cannot make them any stronger.

Selecting Calcium Supplements

Calcium supplements can be found in tablet, liquid, and powder formulations, and are also available in flavored chewable forms. But when you take a trip to your local health food store or pharmacy, remember that all calcium supplements are *not* created equal, so it's important to read labels carefully. The most common forms of calcium supplements are calcium carbonate, calcium citrate, calcium citrate malate, calcium gluconate, and calcium lactate. It can also be found as bone meal and dolomite—the latter being a combination of calcium and magnesium derived from limestone and marble—or as "milk calcium," which is extracted from cow's milk.

Calcium carbonate (found in OsCal and Tums, among others) is one of the most common forms of the mineral found in supplements. Oyster shells are a common source of calcium carbonate, so a label that says "oyster shell calcium" simply means that the product contains calcium carbonate. When this form of calcium comes in contact with stomach acids, it is converted to calcium chloride, which is easily absorbed and used by the body. However, individuals who have low levels of stomach acid may have difficulty absorbing calcium carbonate, and might do better with a calcium citrate supplement, which requires less stomach acidity for absorption. Taking supplements with meals may increase the absorbability of whichever form of calcium you choose.

Calcium citrate and calcium citrate malate are more bioavailable than calcium carbonate. (Bioavailability is the degree to which a nutrient can be used by the body.) However, this advantage is offset somewhat by the fact that—gram for gram of finished product—these forms have less calcium in them, so a larger pill is necessary to get the same amount of calcium. When selecting a calcium supplement, be sure the dose on the bottle refers to the calcium content only, and not to the overall weight of the product. If you have questions about which calcium supplement is best for you, ask your pharmacist for advice.

It's best to stay away from dolomite or bone meal supplements. These supplements contain large amounts of calcium, but can be contaminated with toxins such as lead.

Food Sources

The richest food sources of calcium are dairy products, particularly milk, cheese, and yogurt. Milk is an especially good choice because it's fortified with vitamin D, which is necessary for optimal absorption and utilization of calcium. Other calcium-rich foods include nuts, canned sardines and anchovies (including the bones), and green leafy vegetables, such as collard greens, turnip greens, and mustard greens. You can also look for products that are calcium-fortified, including orange juice, breakfast cereals, and some kinds of bread.

Are You Maximizing Your Calcium Intake?

It's certainly possible to take in the ODA of calcium from dietary sources alone. For example, by drinking three glasses of 1% milk and eating two 8-ounce servings of low-fat yogurt or two 1-ounce servings of cheese, you can easily reach your optimal allowance of this bone-building nutrient. According to statistics, however, most people take in less than half of the ODA of calcium through diet alone. Women take in an average of 639 milligrams of calcium per day, which is less than the average intake of men—even though women have a higher risk of osteoporosis than men. Overall, many men and women could probably benefit from calcium supplementation. Where do you stand?

You can use the information in Table 18.1 to determine your average daily intake of calcium. The foods and beverages included in this table are arranged according to the percentage of the Optimal Daily Allowance of calcium they contain. Start by keeping a food diary for at least three to four days; the longer you keep the diary, the more accurate your calculations will be. Write down everything you eat and drink, as well as the estimated serving size, and refer to the table on page 192 to determine the percentage of the ODA that each food or beverage provides. At the end of each day, add up all of the percentages to see if you've reached 100 percent for the day.

If you find that, on average, you do not take in 100 percent of your ODA of calcium, then you may decide that you want to take mineral supplements for optimal health. But how much of this

Table 18.1. Percent of Calcium ODA in Common Foods and Beverages

Food	Serving Size	Food	Serving Size
5 Percent		Sardines, canned in oil	2 sardines
American cheese	1 ounce	Spinach, boiled	1/2 cup
Anchovies	3 ounces	Tofu	1/2 cup
Beet greens, boiled	1/2 cup	Turnip greens, boiled	1/2 cup
Blue cheese	1 ounce	**10 Percent**	
Broccoli, boiled	1/2 cup	Gruyere cheese	1 ounce
Camembert cheese	1 ounce	Ice milk, vanilla	1 cup
Cheddar cheese	1 ounce	Monterey Jack cheese	1 ounce
Colby cheese	1 ounce	Muenster cheese	1 ounce
Cottage cheese, low-fat	1 cup	Oatmeal, instant	1 packet
Crab, cooked	3 ounces	Provolone cheese	1 ounce
Feta cheese	1 ounce	Pudding, vanilla	1 cup
Figs, dried	10 figs	Rhubarb	1 cup
Garbanzo beans, boiled	1 cup	Swiss cheese	1 ounce
Gouda cheese	1 ounce	**20 Percent**	
Great Northern beans, boiled	1 cup	Macaroni and cheese, homemade	1 cup
Mozzarella cheese	1 ounce	Milk, 1%	1 cup
Navy beans, boiled	1 cup	Ricotta cheese, part-skim	1/2 cup
Pinto beans, boiled	1 cup		
Pizza, homemade	1 slice	Yogurt, low-fat	8 ounces

nutrient do you need to take to reach your ODA? Here's an example of how to perform this calculation: Let's say you determine that you are getting 50 percent (0.50) of your target intake through diet alone. Multiply 0.50 and 1,500 milligrams (the ODA of calcium) and you'll find that you are consuming 750 milligrams of calcium in your diet. To make up the difference, then, you should take in 750 milligrams of calcium in supplement form.

Note that you may not find calcium supplements sold in the exact dose you are looking for. If this is the case, try to come as close as you can to the dose you need without taking several tablets, or splitting pills in half, to get the proper amount. Additionally, you should know that you'll increase your body's calcium absorption by taking half your daily dose in the morning and half in the evening. It's best to take calcium supplements with food, as this also increases absorption.

RECOMMENDATIONS

When it comes to nutrition, there's a lot of important information to remember—so it helps to have what you need to know right at your fingertips. The most critical facts about calcium are summarized below.

What is the Optimal Daily Allowance of calcium?
The ODA of calcium for men and women is 1,500 milligrams. To minimize the risk of developing kidney stones, try to take in as much of the ODA as possible from dietary sources.

What circumstances might affect the amount of calcium you need to take in each day?
Some lifestyle or health factors can affect the amount of calcium you consume or decrease the amount that your body is able to absorb and use. You'll have to be particularly conscientious about taking in the ODA of calcium if:

• You are at risk of vitamin D deficiency.

• You use diuretics.

• You are very physically active.

• You are on a low-calorie diet.

• You eat a diet that's high in protein, fat, fiber, or phosphorus.

• You are pregnant or breast-feeding.

• You are an older person.

Is it possible to consume the optimal amount of calcium through diet alone? By eating a variety of calcium-rich foods, such as dairy products, you can, in fact, reach the ODA of calcium without the need for supplementation. However, many people do not include enough high-calcium foods in their diets. For example, a U.S. Department of Agriculture survey conducted in 1994 found that only 21 percent of women met the RDA of calcium. This is bad news, since women are at an increased risk of osteoporosis in their later years. According to these and other statistics, then, it seems that a lot of men and women would benefit from supplementation.

Chapter 19

Magnesium

The body contains only about 20 to 28 grams of magnesium—
a relatively small quantity, considering that every cell in the
body needs this vital mineral to function. Of this amount,
approximately 60 percent is stored in the bones and teeth; the
remainder is found in the muscles and soft tissues, as well as in the
bloodstream. Magnesium activates over 300 enzymes throughout
the body that are critical for proper cell function, so it's an essential
factor in every major biological process. And now a growing body
of research also suggests that an adequate dietary intake of the
mineral may promote optimal health by helping to maintain normal blood pressure and keeping the heart healthy.

FUNCTIONS IN THE BODY

Magnesium is involved in energy-dependent reactions in the body.
It is essential to the metabolism of glucose, fatty acids, and amino
acids for energy, and plays a part in the use and manufacture of
adenosine triphosphate (ATP), the "energy currency" of the body.
ATP is a compound found in all cells that, when broken down, produces the energy that enables the muscles and other organs to
function.

As mentioned earlier, more than half of the body's supply of
magnesium is contained in the bones and teeth. Along with calcium and phosphorus, the body needs magnesium for bone growth
and to help prevent tooth decay. Experts are exploring the possi-

bility that magnesium supplements may help protect against the development of osteoporosis.

Whereas calcium is important for muscle contraction, magnesium is required for muscle relaxation. When calcium flows into muscle tissue cells, the muscle contracts. When calcium leaves and magnesium replaces it, the muscle relaxes.

In addition to the functions outlined above, magnesium also affects the metabolism of other essential nutrients, such as potassium, calcium, and vitamin D; plays a part in nerve impulse transmission; helps maintain normal heart rhythm; and may also help normalize blood pressure.

HEALTH BENEFITS

Studies have shown that a higher magnesium intake may reduce the risk of heart disease and high blood pressure. And some research has indicated that magnesium supplementation may help save the lives of people who have just had heart attacks, although more studies need to be conducted in this area.

Hypertension

Magnesium helps maintain healthy muscle tone in the blood vessels. Consequently, low magnesium levels in the body may cause the constriction of the muscles in the blood-vessel walls. When the channels in these blood vessels narrow, the result is an increase in blood pressure.

A Japanese study, reported in 1986, observed the effects of supplementation with 600 milligrams of magnesium daily on high blood pressure in twenty-one men. Researchers measured the blood pressure of the participants and the levels of magnesium in their red blood cells at the beginning and end of the four-week study. The results showed that, as magnesium levels increased, both diastolic and systolic blood pressure decreased. (Diastolic is the lowest pressure, when the heart is relaxing; systolic is the highest pressure, during heart contractions.)

In a 1987 study of 615 men of Japanese ancestry, researchers with the Honolulu Heart Study examined the possible association between blood pressure and a variety of nutrients, including magnesium. Of the sixty factors they evaluated, dietary intake of magnesium was most strongly linked to blood pressure control. The researchers reported that the more magnesium the men consumed, the more their blood pressure readings fell.

In 1993, researchers at Umea University Hospital in Sweden conducted a study to determine the effects of magnesium supplements on mild hypertension in seventeen men and women. The participants were divided into two groups: One group took magnesium supplements, while the other group took a placebo, with no active ingredients. The researchers monitored blood pressure of the men and women in both groups over a nine-week period and then reversed the treatments—that is, individuals who at first supplemented with magnesium took a placebo for the next nine weeks, while participants who took a placebo for the first nine weeks switched to magnesium supplements. Systolic and diastolic blood pressure readings were reduced substantially in individuals in both groups when they took magnesium. No significant changes were observed in the groups taking the placebo.

Other studies of the effects of magnesium on high blood pressure have not shown such a high degree of success. For example, a 1991 study at University Hospital in Uppsala, Sweden, showed that magnesium supplementation does not always prove beneficial to people with hypertension. In this study, seventy-one men and women with mild hypertension were divided into two groups, one of which supplemented with magnesium, while the other took a placebo. Over the course of six months, only some of the participants experienced a significant reduction in blood pressure due to magnesium supplements; supplementation with the mineral did not produce any change in the rest of the individuals.

So what's the bottom line? Many experts have concluded that enough evidence has been gathered from existing studies to recommend a magnesium-rich diet for individuals with high blood pressure.

Heart Attack

Although the evidence is not yet conclusive, magnesium may help save the lives of individuals who have just suffered heart attacks. There are two existing theories as to how the nutrient works to improve the outlook for people who have suffered heart attacks. One theory suggests that the mineral relaxes the muscles within the blood vessels, thereby improving blood flow to the heart. The other proposes that magnesium prevents heart muscle cells from suffering further injury.

A 1992 study conducted at Royal Leicester Infirmary in Britain is a good example of how magnesium supplementation may save lives. The study involved more than 2,300 people who had recently suffered heart attacks. One group was given magnesium by injection, while the other group was given a placebo by injection. Individuals in the magnesium group had a 24 percent greater chance of survival during the four-week period after their heart attack than those in the placebo group. Based on these results, the researchers concluded that treatment with magnesium may save an additional twenty-five lives for every thousand heart attack patients treated.

DEFICIENCY SYMPTOMS

Magnesium deficiency is rarely reported among healthy people because the mineral is present in many foods and in drinking water. Severe deficiencies are most often found in individuals whose diets are inadequate or imbalanced, and in people with malabsorption disorders.

The most common symptoms of magnesium deficiency include nausea, muscle weakness or tremors, irritability, loss of appetite, gastrointestinal upset, and rapid heartbeat. Severe deficiency may cause mental changes, including anxiety and nervousness, confusion, depression, and disorientation. In the worst cases, magnesium deficiency may result in coma, although this is very rare.

TOXICITY SYMPTOMS

In most individuals, consuming magnesium in excess of the ODA is not likely to cause harm. However, people with kidney disease are cautioned not to take supplemental magnesium, except with the advice and supervision of a health-care practitioner. Under normal circumstances, the kidneys will cause any extra magnesium to be excreted in the urine. However, in people with kidney

Are You at Risk of Magnesium Deficiency?

How do you know if you're at risk of magnesium deficiency? Take a moment to review the questions below. If you answer yes to any of these questions, you have an above-average risk of developing a deficiency.

❏ *Do you have a parathyroid gland disorder?* The parathyroid gland secretes hormones that help the body maintain adequate levels of magnesium.

❏ *Do you have diabetes?* Diabetes causes an increased loss of magnesium in urine.

❏ *Have you recently suffered a prolonged bout of diarrhea and/or vomiting?* Diarrhea and/or vomiting reduce the amount of magnesium that is available for use by the body.

❏ *Do you use diuretics?* Some diuretics cause an increase in magnesium loss through the kidneys.

❏ *Do you drink large amounts of alcohol?* Alcohol has no real nutritional value. People who abuse alcohol tend to substitute it for nutrient-dense foods, so they generally don't take in adequate amounts of magnesium and other nutrients.

❏ *Are you pregnant or breast-feeding?* Pregnancy is a time of increased nutritional needs because the growth of a new person requires every known nutrient. Extra magnesium is required during pregnancy not only to accommodate for the rapid growth of the developing baby, but also to meet the increased needs of the expectant mother, who may gain 30 pounds or more. According to recent RDAs, pregnant women should take an additional 20 milligrams of magnesium daily. Women who breast-feed require more magnesium to compensate for the average of 30 milligrams of magnesium lost per liter of breast milk. The ODA of magnesium is more than adequate to meet these needs.

disease, excess magnesium can build up in the body and produce toxic symptoms.

Early symptoms of excessive magnesium intake include nausea, vomiting, and low blood pressure. If magnesium levels in the body become extremely high, more serious problems can develop, such as troubled breathing and slow heart rate. In the most severe cases, magnesium toxicity can result in coma and even death, although this happens only rarely.

OPTIMAL DAILY ALLOWANCE

In light of recent studies pointing to magnesium's potential benefits for the heart, as well as its role in normalizing blood pressure, this mineral should be consumed in amounts exceeding the RDA. The Optimal Daily Allowance of magnesium for men and women is 500 milligrams.

Food Sources

Magnesium is found in a wide variety of foods. The richest dietary sources include milk and other dairy products, meat, seafood, nuts (particularly cashews and almonds), legumes, soybeans, leafy green vegetables, and whole-grain cereals. With the exception of bananas, fruits tend to be poor sources of magnesium.

It's important to note that about 80 percent of the magnesium in cereal grains is lost when the germ and outer layers of the grains are removed during milling, so magnesium may be depleted in processed cereals.

Are You Maximizing Your Magnesium Intake?

Most Americans fall short of reaching the ODA of magnesium through diet alone, even though it is, in fact, possible to achieve this intake from food sources. A government study conducted in 1994 found that about 61 percent of adults in the United States regularly failed to reach even the RDA of magnesium. For this reason, it seems clear that the majority of American adults would benefit from supplementation. Where do you stand?

You can use the information in Table 19.1 to determine your average daily intake of magnesium. The foods and beverages included in this table are arranged according to the percentage of the Optimal Daily Allowance of magnesium they contain. Start by keeping a food diary for at least three to four days; the longer you keep the diary, the more accurate your calculations will be. Write down everything you eat and drink, as well as the estimated serving size, and refer to the table on page 202 to determine the percentage of the ODA that each food or beverage provides. At the end of each day, add up all of the percentages to see if you've reached 100 percent for the day.

If you find that, on average, you do not take in 100 percent of your ODA of magnesium, then you may decide that you want to take mineral supplements for optimal health. But how much of this nutrient do you need to take to reach your ODA? Here's an example of how to perform this calculation: Let's say you determine that you're getting 40 percent (0.40) of your target intake through diet alone. Multiply 0.40 and 500 milligrams (the ODA of magnesium) and you'll find that you are consuming 200 milligrams of magnesium in your diet. To make up the difference, then, you should take in 300 milligrams of magnesium in supplement form.

Because magnesium is commonly sold in doses of 250 milligrams, and multivitamin and mineral supplements often supply 100 milligrams of this nutrient, you may have some trouble finding a supplement that contains exactly the amount of magnesium you want. Try to get as close to the ODA as you can without having to take several tablets.

RECOMMENDATIONS

When it comes to nutrition, there's a lot of important information to remember—so it helps to have what you need to know right at your fingertips. The most critical facts about magnesium are summarized below.

What is the Optimal Daily Allowance of magnesium?
The ODA of magnesium for men and women is 500 milligrams.

What circumstances might affect the amount of magnesium you need to take in each day?
Some lifestyle or health factors can affect the amount of magnesium you consume or decrease the amount that your body is able to absorb and use. You'll have to be particularly conscientious about taking in the ODA of magnesium if:

Table 19.1. Percent of Magnesium ODA of Common Foods and Beverages

Food	Serving Size	Food	Serving Size
5 Percent		Pecans	1 ounce
Acorn squash, baked	1/2 cup	Perch	3 ounces
Anchovies	3 ounces	Pineapple juice, canned	1 cup
Artichoke, boiled	1 medium	Pistachio nuts	1 ounce
Banana	1 medium	Potato, baked without skin	1 medium
Beef, top round, broiled	3 1/2 ounces	Prune juice, canned	1 cup
Beet greens, boiled	1/2 cup	Prunes, dried	10 prunes
Beets, boiled	1/2 cup	Raisins, golden, seedless	2/3 cup
Broccoli, boiled	1/2 cup	Scallops	6 large/ 14 small
Buttermilk	1 cup	Sea bass	3 ounces
Butternut squash, boiled	1/2 cup	Sesame seeds	1 tablespoon
Carp	3 ounces	Shrimp	12 large
Carrot juice, canned	6 ounces	Snapper	3 ounces
Chicken breast meat, roasted	1/2 breast	Sole	3 1/2 ounces
leg meat, roasted	1 leg	Spaghetti (enriched), cooked	1 cup
Cod	3 ounces	Tuna, canned in water	3 ounces
Corn, yellow, boiled	1/2 cup	Turkey, light or dark meat, roasted	3 1/2 ounces
Crab, cooked	3 ounces	Yogurt, low-fat	8 ounces
Dates, dried	10 dates	**10 Percent**	
Flounder	3 1/2 ounces	Almonds	1 ounce
Haddock	3 ounces	Avocado	1 medium
Herring	3 ounces	Black-eyed peas, boiled	1 cup
Lobster, cooked	3 ounces	Bran Flakes cereal	1 ounce
Macadamia nuts	1 ounce	Brazil nuts	1 ounce
Milk, 1%	1 cup	Broad beans, boiled	1 cup
Mussels	3 ounces	Cashews	1 ounce
Okra, boiled	1/2 cup	Garbanzo beans, boiled	1 cup
Oysters	6 medium	Great Northern beans, boiled	1 cup
Peanut butter	1 tablespoon		
Peas, green, boiled	1/2 cup		

Food	Serving Size	Food	Serving Size
Halibut	3 ounces	Potato, baked, with skin	1 medium
Hazelnuts	1 ounce	Spinach, boiled	1/2 cup
Kidney beans, boiled	1 cup	Walnuts	1 ounce
Lentils, boiled	1 cup	Wheat germ, toasted	1/4 cup
Lima beans, boiled	1 cup	**20 Percent**	
Mackerel	3 ounces	Black beans, boiled	1 cup
Marinara sauce	1 cup	Figs, dried	10 figs
Miso	1/2 cup	Navy beans, boiled	1 cup
Peaches, dried	10 halves	Sunflower seeds	1 ounce
Peanuts	1 ounce	Tofu	1/2 cup
Pears, dried	10 halves	**30 Percent**	
Pinto beans, boiled	1 cup	Pumpkin seeds	1 ounce

- You have a parathyroid gland disorder.

- You have diabetes.

- You have recently suffered a prolonged bout of diarrhea or vomiting.

- You use diuretics.

- You drink large amounts of alcohol.

- You are pregnant or breast-feeding.

Is it possible to consume the optimal amount of magnesium through diet alone?
It's possible to take in the optimal allowance of magnesium from dietary sources, but government surveys show that the majority of American adults fall short of reaching the optimal allowance. Therefore, it seems clear that most men and women would benefit from supplementation with magnesium.

Chapter 20

Zinc

Although the body contains only 2 to 3 grams of zinc, it is an essential mineral necessary for growth and development. Indeed, deficiency of the nutrient in children may be marked by growth retardation, among other symptoms. Zinc is present in all of the body's cells, although it is most highly concentrated in the eyes, liver, bone, skin, hair, and nails. In men, the nutrient is also concentrated in the prostate and in semen.

In recent years, zinc has been evaluated as an immune system enhancer that may help reduce the frequency of colds and sore throats. Some research has shown that it may shorten the duration of cold symptoms. Additionally, zinc protects the body against the harmful effects of some toxins, such as cadmium and lead.

FUNCTIONS IN THE BODY

One of zinc's most important functions is its involvement in the synthesis of DNA and RNA, the genetic materials contained in all cells. DNA and RNA—collectively called nucleic acids—are necessary for cell division and cell growth, and therefore are essential to reproduction, as well as to the normal growth and development of the human body. Also, the nucleic acids are important for cellular repair, and so they are involved in wound healing. Without adequate amounts of zinc, these processes would be impaired, resulting in some of the common overt deficiency symptoms, including growth retardation, sexual immaturity, and poor wound healing.

Some studies have suggested that zinc is necessary for normal immune system function, and that it may boost the number of white blood cells circulating in the bloodstream. White blood cells help fight infection by acting as the body's first line of defense against foreign "invaders." Zinc deficiency can suppress immunity and can therefore impair the body's defense mechanisms.

Zinc is also part of many enzymes associated with different metabolic processes, including carbohydrate and protein metabolism. As a constituent of the antioxidant enzyme *superoxide dismutase* (SOD), zinc helps to fight and prevent the formation of free radicals, the unstable molecules that have been implicated as the cause of degenerative diseases such as cancer and cardiovascular disease. And zinc acts as a cofactor for the enzyme that allows for the sense of taste.

HEALTH BENEFITS

In 1981, researchers in Belgium conducted a study to determine zinc's effects on immune system function. The study involved fifteen men and women over seventy years of age who took zinc supplements every day for a month, and another group of participants in the same age category who did not supplement with zinc. During the course of the month, doctors closely monitored immune system function in both groups. The results revealed that the group taking zinc supplements had significantly improved in some aspects of their ability to fight disease. For instance, the individuals who supplemented with zinc had more circulating white blood cells, and their antibody response to the tetanus vaccine improved.

A similar study, also conducted in 1981 in Belgium, involved eighty-three men and women who took zinc supplements every day for a month, and a smaller group of twenty men and women who did not take supplemental zinc. During the study, the researchers monitored immune system function in both groups. They found that immune system responses in the participants taking zinc were significantly stronger than were the responses in the control group. The researchers noted that the reaction of white blood cells to foreign substances was enhanced with zinc therapy, while no change was apparent in the group that did not supplement with zinc.

Researchers at the University of Chile's Institute of Nutrition and Food Technology studied the effects of zinc supplementation on thirty-two infants recovering from modest levels of malnutrition. At the beginning of the study, the researchers evaluated the immune system function of each of the infants. Then, over the course of three months, all of the infants were fed the same type of formula, and about half of the total group also received supplemental zinc. When the three months were up, the immune system function of the infants was again evaluated. The results, reported in 1987, clearly showed that immune system function, including the response of white blood cells to foreign substances, improved only in the group that had received zinc supplements. In addition to this, the researchers found that infants with the highest blood-zinc levels ran fevers for the least number of days.

Investigators at the Cleveland Clinic Foundation examined zinc's effects on the common cold in ninety-nine men and women. All of the participants had experienced cold symptoms for less than twenty-four hours at the time they entered the study. The men and women were divided into two groups: One group took zinc gluconate lozenges containing 13.3 milligrams of zinc every two hours while they were awake, while the other group took a placebo. The results? The duration of cold symptoms was reduced by about three days in the participants taking zinc—this group experienced relief of their symptoms in an average of 4.4 days, compared with 7.6 days in the placebo group. The study, which was published in 1996, revealed that nasal congestion and drainage, coughing, hoarseness, and headaches improved more quickly in the participants taking zinc; the relief of other symptoms, including sneezing, fever, and muscle aches, did not differ between the two groups.

DEFICIENCY SYMPTOMS

Signs of zinc deficiency include reduced immune function and greater vulnerability to infections; poor wound healing; loss of appetite; impaired sense of taste and smell; skin rashes; and hair loss. Prolonged deficiency can retard growth in children and can delay the onset of puberty. In pregnant women, deficiency can put the well-being of the fetus at risk because zinc is essential to cell

Are You at Risk of Zinc Deficiency?

How do you know if you're at risk of zinc deficiency? Take a moment to review the questions below. If you answer yes to any of these questions, you have an above-average risk of developing a deficiency.

❏ *Do you use diuretics?* Diuretics cause increased water excretion, and with it, increased losses of zinc from the body.

❏ *Are you a vegetarian?* Vegetarians may be at greater risk of zinc deficiency because they have chosen to avoid eating meat, which is one of the best sources of the mineral. Vegans, who do not eat any animal products, including zinc-rich foods such as milk and eggs, must be even more careful to take in adequate amounts of zinc.

❏ *Is your diet high in fiber?* The fiber in whole grains can interfere with zinc absorption in the intestine. Also, compounds called phytates, which are found primarily in fiber-rich whole grains and beans, bind to zinc and interfere with its absorption.

❏ *Is your diet high in phosphorus- and iron-rich foods?* Although the research is not entirely clear on this point, some studies suggest that these minerals have a mild effect on zinc absorption. (See Chapters 21 and 23 for foods that are high in phosphorus and iron.)

❏ *Do you drink large amounts of alcohol?* Alcohol interferes with the body's absorption of zinc because it accelerates loss of the mineral in the urine. Also, alcoholics tend to substitute alcohol—which has no real nutritional value—for nutrient-dense foods, so they generally don't take in enough zinc and other nutrients.

❏ *Are you pregnant or breast-feeding?* Pregnancy is a time of increased nutritional needs because the growth of a new person requires every known nutrient. In animal studies, zinc deficiency has been associated with developmental disorders in the young. Mothers who breast-feed should also be careful to take in extra zinc to compensate for the 1.5 milligrams per liter that are lost through breast milk. The National Research Council has recommended an additional 7 milligrams of zinc daily for breast-feeding mothers. The ODA of zinc is more than adequate to meet these needs.

❏ *Are you an older person?* Many older people have poor dietary habits, usually because they are on limited budgets or they live alone and do not cook much for themselves.

division and cell growth, and therefore to the growth and development of the baby.

People with sickle-cell anemia are particularly prone to deficiency. In sickle-cell anemia, the red blood cells contain abnormal hemoglobin, which causes the cells to become crescent- or sickle-shaped. These deformed cells are very fragile, and they break up as they travel through blood vessels. Red blood cells are rich in zinc, so when they break apart, zinc is released from the cells and lost from the body through the urine.

Finally, zinc deficiency is more common in populations whose zinc intake is derived primarily from grain sources because these foods contain zinc-binding substances called *phytates*. Phytates attach themselves to zinc and block its absorption by the body.

TOXICITY SYMPTOMS

Zinc generally causes toxic symptoms only when taken in large amounts, such as 2,000 milligrams or more taken at one time, or a slightly smaller dosage taken regularly over the course of several weeks. Signs of zinc toxicity at this intake level usually include vomiting and diarrhea. High dosages of zinc—150 to 450 milligrams—taken regularly for prolonged periods may interfere with immune function in much the same way that zinc deficiency can impair immunity.

Interestingly, excessive intake of zinc, as little as two times the ODA of 15 milligrams, can lower the body's copper content and may even cause a marginal copper deficiency. This is potentially harmful, since copper aids in the formation of bone, hemoglobin, and red blood cells, and is also essential to the formation of collagen.

OPTIMAL DAILY ALLOWANCE

The Optimal Daily Allowance of zinc is 15 milligrams. Women who are breast-feeding should take in 19 milligrams daily to compensate for the amount of the mineral that is lost in breast milk.

Food Sources

The best sources of zinc are red meat, poultry, liver, fish and other seafood (most notably raw oysters), egg yolks, and legumes. Remember that the zinc contained in whole grains is not always readily available for use by the body. The fiber in whole grains can interfere with zinc absorption in the intestine, and phytates bind to zinc and block its absorption.

The amount of zinc contained in plants depends to some degree on the soil in which the plants were grown, specifically on the zinc concentrations in that soil. Despite the fact that zinc is available in common foods, research shows that many people do not get enough zinc from their diets.

Are You Maximizing Your Zinc Intake?

According to government surveys, American men and women do not take in even the RDA of zinc through diet alone, so we can surmise that even fewer adults achieve the ODA. And while it *is* possible to reach the ODA from dietary sources, you would have to eat ten 8-ounce servings of low-fat yogurt, 10 cups of Manhattan clam chowder, or more than 11 ounces of beef brisket! Most people will have to rely on supplements to take in the optimal allowance of zinc. Where do you stand?

You can use the information in Table 20.1 to determine your average daily intake of zinc. The foods and beverages included in this table are arranged according to the percentage of the Optimal Daily Allowance of zinc they contain. Remember that the ODA of zinc is 15 milligrams for all adults; breast-feeding women should aim to take in 19 milligrams daily. For this self-test, we'll use 15 milligrams.

Start by keeping a food diary for at least three to four days; the longer you keep the diary, the more accurate your calculations will be. Write down everything you eat and drink, as well as the estimated serving size, and refer to the table on page 211 to determine the percentage of the ODA that each food or beverage provides. At the end of each day, add up all of the percentages to see if you've reached 100 percent for the day. (If your ODA falls elsewhere in the range, remember to take that into account when calculating your percentages.)

If you find that, on average, you do not take in 100 percent of your ODA of zinc, then you may decide that you want to take

Table 20.1. Percent of Zinc ODA in Common Foods and Beverages

Food	Serving Size	Food	Serving Size
5 Percent		Perch	3 ounces
Almonds	1 ounce	Provolone cheese	1 ounce
American cheese	1 ounce	Scallops	6 large/ 14 small
Anchovies	3 ounces	Shrimp	12 large
Blue cheese	1 ounce	Sunflower seeds	1 ounce
Brazil nuts	1 ounce	Swiss cheese	1 ounce
Buttermilk	1 cup	Swordfish	3 ounces
Carp	3 ounces	Tofu	$1/2$ cup
Cheddar cheese	1 ounce	Walnuts	1 ounce
Chicken breast meat, roasted light meat only, roasted thigh meat, roasted	$1/2$ breast $3\,1/2$ ounces 1 thigh	**10 Percent**	
		Beef soup, chunky	1 cup
Chicken soup, chunky	1 cup	Black beans, boiled	1 cup
Clams	4 large/ 9 small	Black-eyed peas, boiled	1 cup
		Broad beans, boiled	1 cup
Colby cheese	1 ounce	Cashews	1 ounce
Cottage cheese, low-fat	1 cup	Chicken light and dark meat, roasted leg meat, roasted	$3\,1/2$ ounces 1 leg
Egg	1 large	Green Northern beans, boiled	1 cup
Feta cheese	1 ounce		
Frankfurter, beef	1 frank	Ham, canned	$3\,1/2$ ounces
Gouda cheese	1 ounce	Kidney beans, boiled	1 cup
Herring	3 ounces	Lentils, boiled	1 cup
Ice cream, vanilla	1 cup	Lima beans, boiled	1 cup
Milk, 1%	1 cup	Lobster, cooked	3 ounces
Monterey Jack cheese	1 ounce	Manhattan clam chowder	1 cup
Muenster cheese	1 ounce	Navy beans, boiled	1 cup
Mussels	3 ounces	Pecans	1 ounce
Oatmeal, instant	1 packet	Pinto beans, boiled	1 cup
Peanuts	1 ounce	Pork loin, roasted	$3\,1/2$ ounces
Peas, green, boiled	$1/2$ cup		

Food	Serving Size	Food	Serving Size
Pumpkin seeds	1 ounce	**30 Percent**	
Ricotta cheese, part-skim	½ cup	Beef bottom round, braised brisket, braised flank steak, broiled ground (lean), baked top round, broiled	3½ ounces 3½ ounces 3½ ounces 3½ ounces 3½ ounces
Turkey, light and dark meat, roasted	3½ ounces		
Yogurt, low-fat	8 ounces	Corned beef, cooked	3½ ounces
20 Percent		Miso	½ cup
Chicken liver, simmered	3½ ounces	Wheat germ, toasted	¼ cup
Crab, cooked	3 ounces	**90 Percent**	
Pork shoulder, roasted	3½ ounces	Oysters, Pacific	6 medium
Turkey, dark meat only, roasted	3½ ounces	**100 Percent or More**	
Vegetable soup, chunky	1 cup	Oysters, Atlantic	6 medium

mineral supplements for optimal health. But how much of this nutrient do you need to take to reach your ODA? Here's an example of how to perform this calculation: Let's say you determine that you're getting 20 percent (0.20) of your target intake through diet alone. Multiply 0.20 and 15 milligrams (the ODA of zinc) and you'll find that you are consuming 3 milligrams of zinc in your diet. To make up the difference, then, you should take in 12 milligrams of zinc in supplement form. Many multivitamin and mineral supplements contain 15 milligrams of zinc; combined with dietary sources, this amount is enough to meet everyone's needs.

RECOMMENDATIONS

When it comes to nutrition, there's a lot of important information to remember—so it helps to have what you need to know right at your fingertips. The most critical facts about zinc are summarized below.

What is the Optimal Daily Allowance of zinc?
The ODA of zinc for men and women is 15 milligrams. Women who are breast-feeding should take in 19 milligrams of zinc per day.

What circumstances might affect the amount of zinc you need to take in each day?

Some lifestyle or health factors can affect the amount of zinc you consume or decrease the amount that your body is able to absorb and use. You'll have to be particularly conscientious about taking in the ODA of zinc if:

- You use diuretics.

- You are a vegetarian.

- Your diet is high in fiber or in phosphorus- and iron-rich foods.

- You drink large amounts of alcohol.

- You are pregnant or breast-feeding.

- You are an older person.

Is it possible to consume the optimal amount of zinc through diet alone?

According to government surveys, the majority of American adults do not take in even the RDA of zinc, much less the ODA. Furthermore, while it's possible to take in the ODA from dietary sources, it may be difficult to achieve these intakes. As such, most men and women will probably benefit from supplementation.

Chapter 21

Iron

Of all the essential minerals, the most widely known may be iron. It is required by every cell in the body because of the important part it plays in oxygen transport. Iron is also present in a number of enzymes that are involved in the production of energy.

About 75 percent of the body's iron is present in hemoglobin, the oxygen-carrying protein found in red blood cells. An additional 5 percent is part of another protein substance called *myoglobin*, which stores oxygen reserves in muscle tissue. Iron is also stored in the bone marrow, liver, and spleen in the form of *ferritin* and *hemosiderin*, which are protein-iron complexes that serve as iron reserves.

FUNCTIONS IN THE BODY

The most important function of iron is to help hemoglobin transport oxygen through the bloodstream to all of the body's cells. Iron is also present in a variety of enzymes that are essential to the production of energy. Enzymes are catalysts that initiate or speed chemical reactions in the body. A number of these iron-containing enzymes require iron to use oxygen in energy pathways.

DEFICIENCY SYMPTOMS

Despite the careful guarding of iron stores by the body, iron deficiency is the single most common nutrient deficiency in the United

States and the world. This is due to a number of factors, chief among them inadequate iron intake, either from lack of food or from too much of the wrong foods. Vegetarians are especially susceptible to iron deficiency because foods that are highest in iron—meat, poultry, and fish—are excluded from their diets. Vegans are at greater risk because they do not eat any animal products, including eggs and milk, which are also rich sources of iron.

Blood loss is a primary nonnutritional cause of deficiency, because such a large percentage of the body's iron is contained in the blood. Menstruating women may be at risk because some amount of iron is lost each month; for women whose menstrual periods are especially heavy, losses are particularly significant. Gastrointestinal bleeding (such as from ulcers) can also cause blood loss that may lead to iron deficiency, and bleeding during and after surgery or as the result of an injury is a risk factor for deficiency, as well.

Severe iron deficiency is known as *hypochromic microcytic anemia,* or iron-deficiency anemia. With this form of anemia, the amount of hemoglobin in each red blood cell declines, reducing the oxygen-carrying capacity of the cell. The red blood cells are smaller than normal and are also pale in color. Because the hemoglobin content of the blood may be significantly reduced, the body's tissues become starved for oxygen, producing a diverse group of symptoms.

Babies and young children who have iron-deficiency anemia are usually pale, irritable and restless, and are often fatigued. Some studies have also shown that iron-deficient children have short attention spans. Adults who have this form of anemia tire easily, and may feel listless and irritable. Other symptoms experienced by iron-deficient adults include: headaches, shortness of breath, decreased appetite, and increased susceptibility to infections and illnesses. In the worst cases, iron-deficiency anemia can result in heart attack or stroke because the oxygen needs of vital organs are not met.

TOXICITY SYMPTOMS

Individuals who are in good health run little risk of experiencing side effects from high intakes of iron—even up to 75 milligrams

Are You at Risk of Iron Deficiency?

How do you know if you're at risk of iron deficiency? Take a moment to review the questions below. If you answer yes to any of these questions, you have an above-average risk of developing a deficiency.

❏ *Have you lost blood recently?* Gastrointestinal bleeding may occur in conditions such as certain cancers, hemorrhoids, colitis, and ulcers, and can also be caused by aspirin and other non-steroidal anti-inflammatory drugs (NSAIDs). Blood loss significant enough to cause iron deficiency may also occur during and after surgery, during childbirth, or as the result of an injury.

❏ *Are you menstruating?* The average woman loses 15 to 30 milligrams of iron each month during menstruation; for women whose menstrual periods are very heavy or last for a long time, losses are significantly higher. For this reason, women who have not yet reached menopause require more iron each day than men or older women.

❏ *Do you donate blood often?* You may be increasing your risk of developing iron deficiency if you donate to a blood bank, because some amount of iron is lost in every pint of donated blood.

❏ *Are you a vegetarian, or is your diet low in animal protein?* Vegetables, beans, and grains contain nonheme iron, which is not absorbed as easily by the body as the iron in meat. People who eat little or no animal protein should make sure they take in adequate vitamin C to enhance the absorption of nonheme iron.

❏ *Are you pregnant?* Pregnancy is a time of increased nutritional needs because the growth of a new person requires every known nutrient. Iron is important during pregnancy because the developing fetus draws upon its mother's iron stores.

In addition to the factors noted above, iron deficiency can be caused by poor absorption of the iron in foods. Tea, coffee, soy protein, wheat bran, calcium supplements, and fiber can interfere with iron absorption. Antacids also impair iron availability by altering the pH of the intestines.

per day—from dietary and/or supplemental sources. That's because the body has a built-in mechanism to protect itself against iron overload; the mucous lining in the intestine decreases iron absorption when excessive amounts of iron are taken in.

Children, however, are at particularly high risk of iron toxicity. Sadly, thousands of cases of iron poisoning occur each year in youngsters, often after children swallow their parents' iron pills or multimineral supplements. Even a dose as small as 3 grams can be fatal for a child; for adults, a fatal dose is estimated to be nearly eighty times higher.

Hemochromatosis is a rare and potentially deadly hereditary condition in which the mucous lining of the intestine fails to regulate iron absorption, so the body accumulates and stores excess iron. This causes a buildup of extra iron in the tissues of many

---

How Risky Is Excess Iron Intake?

There is much debate surrounding the issue of whether excess iron is linked to coronary heart disease. The results of some studies have shown that high blood levels of iron are likely to cause heart disease. For example, in 1992, researchers at the University of Kuopio, Finland, showed that excess iron in the body increases the risk of heart attack. In fact, according to this study, only cigarette smoking was more likely to lead to heart problems in men.

During the three-year Finnish study, which involved nearly 2,000 participants, men with blood ferritin levels of 200 micrograms per liter or greater were more than twice as likely to have a heart attack than men with lower levels. Men who had both high blood levels of iron and high levels of "bad" low-density lipoprotein (LDL) cholesterol were more than four times as likely to have a heart attack, compared with men who had low levels of both iron and LDL cholesterol.

The results of this study seem to provide support for a theory proposed by Veterans Administration pathologist Jerome Sullivan in the early 1980s. He suggested that the monthly loss of iron during menstruation might protect premenopausal women from heart disease. According to Sullivan's theory, postmenopausal women have an increased risk of heart disease that corresponds

organs, which can damage the liver, heart, pancreas, and spleen, and can also accumulate to toxic levels in the bone marrow. The end result may be serious health problems such as cirrhosis and irregular heart rhythm. Men are more likely to be affected by hemochromatosis because their bodies do not eliminate excess iron.

OPTIMAL DAILY ALLOWANCE

The Optimal Daily Allowance of iron is lower for men than it is for premenopausal women. Men should take in 10 milligrams of iron daily, whereas women who have not reached menopause should aim for 15 milligrams daily for optimal health. For women whose menstrual periods are especially heavy, the ODA of iron is 20 milligrams. Because postmenopausal women no longer lose substan-

with increased levels of iron in the body after menstruation has ceased permanently. Few researchers took this hypothesis seriously—until the Finnish study was published.

Although more recent research has raised doubts about the study conducted at the University of Kuopio, the final word is certainly not in on this issue. In fact, a study published in April 1994 by the Center for Health Statistics of the Centers for Disease Control and Prevention found contradictory evidence about the relationship between iron levels in the body and the risk of coronary heart disease. For this study, which began in the early 1970s, more than 4,500 men and women gave blood samples that were used to measure body iron stores. Researchers monitored the health of the participants until 1987 to determine whether high iron levels were associated with an increased risk of heart disease. In this study, iron levels were *not* linked with heart disease. In fact, in a somewhat surprising finding, the study indicated that iron has a *protective* effect against heart disease.

Future studies should help clarify this issue. For now, it seems best to obtain most of your daily recommendation for iron from food sources, and to supplement this intake—if necessary—with low-dose iron tablets. Only people with medical problems that cause chronic above-average loss of blood should take high-level supplements.

tial amounts of iron each month, their requirement for the mineral is equal to that of men: 10 milligrams daily.

The amount of iron needed to treat iron-deficiency anemia is much higher than the intake needed to maintain optimal health. A typical daily recommendation for an individual who has iron-deficiency anemia may include three 50- to 100-milligram tablets of elemental iron, often taken with vitamin C supplements to enhance absorption. Note, however, that this high level should be taken *only until the deficiency is corrected,* to avoid the risk of iron overload. If you think that you may have iron-deficiency anemia, it is not advisable to begin self-treatment. Schedule an appointment with your health-care practitioner to make sure that the diagnosis is indeed iron-deficiency anemia. He or she will be able to guide you if you need to take high-level doses of supplemental iron. Occasionally, oral iron supplements do not eliminate the symptoms of iron deficiency. If this is the case, your doctor will probably recommend injections to bring your iron levels up to normal.

Food Sources

Red meat and liver are the best food sources of iron; however, you should not rely heavily on these foods for your iron intake because they are high in saturated fat and cholesterol. Poultry and fish are good iron-rich animal foods to select, rather than fatty meats. Other excellent sources of iron are dark green leafy vegetables, peas, corn, beans, dried fruits, prunes, raisins, and eggs. In addition, many breakfast cereals, breads, and pastas are iron-fortified.

Remember that the body absorbs heme iron more easily than the nonheme form of iron. Heme iron is found in animal foods, including meats, liver, chicken, and fish. Nonheme iron is the form of the mineral present in plant foods, such as dried fruits, nuts, legumes, and whole grains. To enhance the absorption of nonheme iron, try to eat foods that are rich in heme iron at the same meal, or take vitamin C. Vegetarians need to be especially careful to take measures to increase iron absorption, since their diets contain very few sources of heme iron, and instead include a wide variety of vegetables, legumes, and grains.

It's interesting to note that cooking foods in an iron skillet can actually increase their iron content. That's because some ferric iron from the metal pan is absorbed into the food while it's cooking. Although this form of iron is not absorbed as well as the heme iron contained in red meat, some does get into the body.

Are You Maximizing Your Iron Intake?

It is possible to consume the ODA of iron through diet alone, but evidence suggests that few people actually take in the optimal allowance. Although iron supplements are appropriate when your diet does not supply the amounts you need, you must exercise caution to avoid the possibility of iron overload.

You can use the information in Table 21.1 to determine your average daily intake of iron. The foods and beverages included in this table are arranged according to the percentage of the Optimal Daily Allowance of iron they contain. The ODA for men and postmenopausal women is 10 milligrams per day; for younger women, it is 15 milligrams daily, up to 20 milligrams for women with heavy menstrual flow. For this self-test, we'll use the mid-range ODA, 15 milligrams.

Start by keeping an accurate food diary for at least three to four days; the longer you keep the diary, the more accurate your calculations will be. Write down everything you eat and drink, as well as the estimated serving size, and refer to the table on page 222 to determine the percentage of the ODA that each food or beverage provides. At the end of each day, add up all of the percentages to see if you've reached 100 percent for the day.

If you find that, on average, you do not take in 100 percent of your ODA of iron, then you may decide that you want to take mineral supplements for optimal health. But how much of this nutrient do you need to take to reach your ODA? Here's an example of how to perform this calculation: Let's say you determine that you're getting 60 percent (0.60) of your target intake through diet alone. Multiply 0.60 and 15 milligrams (the ODA of iron) and you'll find that you are consuming 9 milligrams of iron in your diet. To make up the difference, then, you should take in 6 milligrams of iron in supplement form.

Many supplements contain anywhere from 15 to 18 milligrams of iron, so you can easily meet the ODA by taking only one pill—

Table 21.1. Percent of Iron ODA in Common Foods and Beverages

Food	Serving Size	Food	Serving Size
5 Percent		Tortilla, corn	1 tortilla
Acorn squash, baked	1/2 cup	Turkey, light meat, roasted	3 1/2 ounces
Almonds	1 ounce		
Apple juice, canned	1 cup	Vegetable soup	1 cup
Avocado, California	1/2 medium	**10 Percent**	
Bagel	1 bagel	Anchovies	3 ounces
Beet greens, boiled	1/2 cup	Artichoke, boiled	1 medium
Brazil nuts	1 ounce	Beef	
Broccoli, boiled	1/2 cup	brisket, braised	3 1/2 ounces
		flank steak, braised	3 1/2 ounces
Brussels sprouts, boiled	4 sprouts	ground (lean), baked	3 1/2 ounces
		top round, braised	3 1/2 ounces
Carp	3 ounces	Beef soup	1 cup
Chicken		Broad beans, boiled	1 cup
breast meat, roasted	1/2 breast	Cashews	1 ounce
leg meat, roasted	1 leg		
light and dark meat, roasted	3 1/2 ounces	Corn Flakes cereal	1 cup
		Corned beef, cooked	3 1/2 ounces
Chicken soup	1 cup	Manhattan clam chowder	1 cup
Dates, dried	10 dates	Marinara sauce	1 cup
Egg	1 large	Pistachio nuts	1 ounce
Haddock	3 ounces	Potato, baked, with skin	1 medium
Ham, canned	3 1/2 ounces	Prunes, dried	10 prunes
Hazel nuts	1 ounce	Raisins, seedless	2/3 cup
Herring	3 ounces	Rice, white (enriched), cooked	1 cup
Lamb			
loin chop, broiled	1 chop	Shrimp	12 large
leg of, roasted	3 ounces	Spaghetti (enriched)	1 cup
Mackerel	3 ounces	Sunflower seeds	1 ounce
Peanuts	1 ounce	Trout	3 ounces
Peas, green, boiled	1/2 cup	Tuna, canned in water	3 ounces
Pita bread pocket	1 pita	Turkey, dark meat, roasted	3 1/2 ounces
Pudding, chocolate	1 cup		
Rice, brown, cooked	1 cup	Wheat germ, toasted	1/4 cup

Food	Serving Size	Food	Serving Size
20 Percent		Navy beans, boiled	1 cup
Beef, bottom round, braised	3½ ounces	Oysters	6 medium
		40 Percent	
Black beans, boiled	1 cup	Beef liver, braised	3½ ounces
Black-eyed peas, boiled	½ cup	Lentils, boiled	1 cup
Figs, dried	10 figs	Oatmeal, instant	1 packet
Great Northern beans, boiled	1 cup	Tofu	½ cup
Mussels	3 ounces	**50 Percent**	
Pinto beans, boiled	1 cup	Chicken liver, simmered	3½ ounces
Prune juice	1 cup	Cream of Wheat, instant	1 packet
Pumpkin seeds	1 ounce	**70 Percent**	
Spinach, boiled	½ cup	Clams	4 large or 9 small
30 Percent			
Garbanzo beans, boiled	½ cup	**100 Percent or More**	
Kidney beans, boiled	1 cup	Breakfast cereals (enriched)	1 cup
Lima beans, boiled	1 cup		

without the risk of iron overload. It's best to take iron supplements with food or a glass of juice.

RECOMMENDATIONS

When it comes to nutrition, there's a lot of important information to remember—so it helps to have what you need to know right at your fingertips. The most critical facts about iron are summarized below.

What is the Optimal Daily Allowance of iron?
The ODA of iron for men and postmenopausal women is 10 milligrams. Premenopausal women should take in 15 milligrams per day to compensate for the amount of iron lost during menstruation. For women who experience heavy bleeding during menstruation, the ODA is 20 milligrams.

What circumstances might affect the amount of iron you need to take in each day?

Some lifestyle or health factors can affect the amount of iron you consume or decrease the amount that your body is able to absorb and use. You'll have to be particularly conscientious about taking in the ODA of iron if:

- You have lost blood recently.

- You are menstruating.

- You donate blood often.

- You eat little or no animal protein.

- You are pregnant.

Is it possible to consume the optimal amount of iron through diet alone?

While it's possible to take in the ODA of iron from dietary sources alone, most people do not reach their optimal intake. Therefore, iron supplements may be beneficial. It's important to remember, however, that you need to be very careful about taking supplements because of the risk of iron overload.

Chapter 22

Selenium

Selenium is a late bloomer among the minerals—it wasn't classified as a nutrient essential to human health until 1979. Even then, a Recommended Dietary Allowance (RDA) was not established for this mineral for more than a decade. Today, selenium is widely regarded in the scientific community as a potentially powerful antioxidant, and research suggests that it may be an important protective agent against heart disease and some forms of cancer.

FUNCTIONS IN THE BODY

Selenium, in conjunction with an enzyme called *glutathione peroxidase*, helps prevent oxidative damage in the body. As you will remember from Chapter 3, antioxidants neutralize harmful, unstable molecules called free radicals. Glutathione peroxidase, with the aid of selenium and vitamin E, protects the body against free radicals and helps prevent damage to the body's tissues, cells, and molecules. By consuming adequate amounts of both selenium and vitamin E, you can help protect your body against the kind of cellular damage that is believed to contribute to several serious diseases.

In addition to its antioxidant function, selenium protects the body against the toxic effects of mercury, copper, and arsenic, apparently by binding to these substances to render them less harmful.

HEALTH BENEFITS

Ongoing research into the effects of selenium has concentrated in two areas: cancer and heart disease. Findings indicate that selenium might help prevent both conditions.

Cancer

Some studies have suggested that selenium deficiency contributes to cancer, and there is evidence that selenium may help prevent cancer. However, while many findings have been positive, the research has produced conflicting findings, overall.

As part of a large, multicenter study at universities throughout the United States, blood samples were collected from nearly 11,000 men and women. Over the course of the next five years, 111 of the participants were diagnosed with cancer. When blood samples from the individuals with cancer were compared with blood samples from 210 cancer-free men and women, researchers found that blood selenium levels were substantially lower in the people with cancer. Specifically, individuals with selenium concentrations in the lowest one-fifth of the group were twice as likely to develop cancer as men and women in the highest one-fifth. Cancers of the gastrointestinal tract and prostate cancer were most strongly linked to low blood levels of selenium.

In 1984, investigators at the University of Kuopio in Finland reported the findings of their study examining a possible link between selenium and cancer. As part of the study, more than 8,000 men and women were interviewed and filled out health and life-style questionnaires. The participants also gave blood samples, which were frozen for future study. During the next six years, 128 of the men and women involved in the study were diagnosed with cancer. When blood samples of the 128 individuals with cancer were compared with blood samples from 128 cancer-free men and women, the investigators discovered that blood selenium levels were significantly lower in participants who developed cancer. In fact, individuals with the lowest levels of selenium had three times the risk of developing cancer—particularly of the gastrointestinal tract and of the blood—when compared with people who had higher blood levels of selenium.

Another study of selenium's effects on cancer, conducted in the

Netherlands, involved more than 120,000 men and women who completed dietary questionnaires and provided toenail clippings for researchers to determine their selenium levels. Over the next three years, 155 of the participants developed stomach cancer, 313 were diagnosed with colon cancer, and 166 contracted rectal cancer. While evidence did not conclusively indicate that selenium protected any of the participants from either colon or rectal cancer, the research seemed to suggest that higher selenium levels actually reduced the risk of stomach cancer, particularly for men. The results, published in 1993, revealed that men ranking in the highest one-fifth for selenium levels had a 36 percent lower risk of developing stomach cancer, compared with men in the lowest one-fifth of the group.

A separate study, published in 1996, looked at the effects of supplemental selenium on the development of cancer in more than 1,300 men and women, eighteen to eighty years old, who had all previously had either basal cell or squamous cell skin cancer. One group of participants took 200 micrograms of supplemental selenium daily, while the rest of the individuals took a placebo, with no active ingredients. The results of the study showed that selenium supplements did not reduce the number of new cases of skin cancer; however, supplementation was, in fact, associated with a decline in the incidence of other forms of cancer. Researchers found that the group taking selenium had a 37 percent reduction in the overall incidence of cancer and a 50 percent decrease in total cancer deaths. More specifically, participants supplementing with selenium had 63 percent fewer cases of prostate cancer, 58 percent fewer colorectal cancers, and 46 percent fewer lung cancers than the placebo group. There was no significant difference in the incidence of other types of cancer, including cancers of the breast, bladder, head, and neck.

In contrast to the research described above, the results of other studies have shown that selenium does not appear to have an effect on the incidence of cancer. As part of the Nurses' Health Study at Harvard Medical School in Massachusetts, beginning in 1982, more than 62,000 nurses provided toenail clippings to researchers, who used the clippings to determine the women's selenium levels. Over the course of the next four and a half years, 434 of the participants were diagnosed with breast cancer. The researchers found that selenium levels of the women with breast cancer were similar to levels in women who did not have cancer—an indication that selenium may not afford protection against breast cancer.

Cardiovascular Disease

Promising research has revealed that selenium may provide protection against cardiovascular disease. In a study that began in 1972 in Finland, researchers froze blood samples obtained from more than 11,000 men and women, and then closely monitored the health of the participants during the next seven years. Over the course of the study, 367 of the participants developed cardiovascular disease; of those individuals, 170 subsequently died from the disease. When blood samples from the individuals with cardiovascular disease were compared with samples from people who did not develop the disease, researchers found that those who remained healthy had higher selenium levels. The results of the study revealed that individuals with very low levels of selenium were about three times more likely to die of coronary heart disease and twice as likely to suffer a heart attack as people with high levels.

To further determine selenium's effects on cardiovascular disease, researchers at Creighton University School of Medicine in Omaha, Nebraska, measured the blood selenium levels of ninety-one men and women with chest pain. The individuals involved in the study then underwent a procedure called *arteriography,* in which X-rays were taken of their coronary arteries to determine the presence and extent of the heart disease. In 1984, the researchers reported that participants with lower selenium levels had more severe cases of coronary disease. In cases where two or three of the arteries supplying blood to the heart were affected by the disease, these individuals had significantly lower selenium levels than participants who did not have any apparent coronary artery disease.

In a 1990 study conducted at the University of Auckland, New Zealand, researchers measured blood selenium levels of 252 men and women who had recently had heart attacks. The blood levels of selenium in the individuals who had heart attacks were then compared with blood selenium levels in 838 healthy individuals. Participants who had experienced heart attacks had blood levels of selenium that were about 6 percent lower than the measurements of their healthy counterparts. Men in the lower half of the group for selenium had a 60 percent greater risk of having a heart attack than did men in the higher half. Women in the lower half of the group had a 70 percent higher risk than did women in the higher half of the group.

DEFICIENCY SYMPTOMS

The most obvious symptoms of selenium deficiency include muscular weakness and discomfort. In the most serious cases, a long-term deficiency may increase the risk of cardiovascular disease and heart attack, as well as cancers of the lung, breast, and urinary and gastrointestinal tracts.

In 1979, researchers described an association between selenium

---

Are You at Risk of Selenium Deficiency?

How do you know if you're at risk of selenium deficiency? Take a moment to review the questions below. If you answer yes to any of these questions, you have an above-average risk of developing a deficiency.

❏ *Are you under physical or emotional stress?* Some animal studies have shown that any type of physical or emotional stress on the body can contribute to selenium deficiencies.

❏ *Is your diet low in vitamin E?* To some degree, the roles of selenium and vitamin E overlap in the body, and it's possible to make up for a deficiency in one of these nutrients by consuming more of the other.

❏ *Are you pregnant or breast-feeding?* Pregnancy is a time of increased nutritional needs because the growth of a new person requires every known nutrient. According to the National Research Council, pregnant women should take in an additional 10 micrograms of selenium daily. Also, because about 15 to 20 micrograms of selenium are lost in every liter of breast milk, women who breast-feed are advised to take in an additional 20 micrograms per day of selenium. The ODA of selenium is more than adequate to meet these needs.

deficiency and a heart-muscle condition called *Keshan disease*, also known as *cardiomyopathy*. The disease was first identified in the Keshan province of China, an area of the country with selenium-deficient soils. Keshan disease, which primarily affects children and women in their childbearing years, is now known to cause enlargement of the heart muscle and, eventually, heart failure.

TOXICITY SYMPTOMS

Reports of selenium toxicity are rare, and usually occur in individuals who take far in excess of the recommended dosage of the mineral. According to one study, an individual experienced symptoms after taking 1 milligram daily over a two-year period. In another incident, a manufacturer mistakenly produced supplements containing 27 milligrams of selenium per tablet. More than a dozen cases of toxicity were reported due to this error.

Too much selenium in the body can cause symptoms such as nausea, abdominal pain, diarrhea, fatigue, irritability, and hair and nail damage. A garlic-like odor on the breath may also become apparent.

OPTIMAL DAILY ALLOWANCE

Conclusive evidence of the need for selenium has emerged only in recent years, and scientists are still learning about the mineral's functions in the body. To date, research has indicated that higher selenium intakes may help prevent cardiovascular disease and some forms of cancer.

The Optimal Daily Allowance of selenium for all adults is 200 micrograms, which is higher than the current RDA. Be aware, however, that there's no evidence that amounts higher than the ODA will confer additional benefits.

Food Sources

The best sources of selenium are seafood, organ meats, muscle meats, whole grains such as whole wheat and oats, cashews, kidney beans, mushrooms, and onions. However, the selenium content of foods like grains and vegetables is dependent upon the selenium content of the soils in which the foods were grown, and the selenium content of the water used to nourish them.

Are You Maximizing Your Selenium Intake?

According to one survey, the average American adult takes in about 108 micrograms of selenium per day. While this amount is well above the RDA, it is still below the Optimal Daily Allowance. In areas of the country where the selenium content of the soil is especially poor, many people fall even farther below those levels. It seems clear that most people would benefit from selenium supplements. Where do you stand?

You can use the information in Table 22.1 to determine your average daily intake of selenium. The foods and beverages included in this table are arranged according to the percentage of the Optimal Daily Allowance of selenium they contain. Start by keeping a food diary for at least three to four days; the longer you keep the diary, the more accurate your calculations will be. Write down everything you eat and drink, as well as the estimated serving size, and refer to the table on page 232 to determine the percentage of the ODA that each food or beverage provides. At the end of each day, add up all of the percentages to see if you've reached 100 percent for the day.

If you find that, on average, you do not take in 100 percent of your ODA of selenium, then you may decide that you want to take mineral supplements for optimal health. But how much of this nutrient do you need to take to reach your ODA? Here's an example of how to perform this calculation: Let's say you determine that you're getting 60 percent (0.60) of your target intake through diet alone. Multiply 0.60 and 200 micrograms (the ODA of selenium) and you'll find that you are consuming 120 micrograms of selenium in your diet. To make up the difference, then, you should take in 80 micrograms of selenium in supplement form.

Because selenium is commonly sold in doses of 50 or 100 micrograms, you may have some trouble finding a supplement that contains the exact amount that you want of the mineral. If you need a supplement of 40 micrograms, it's fine to go a little higher and take a 50-microgram tablet. This is more than adequate to meet your needs without any health risks.

Table 22.1. Percent of Selenium ODA in Common Foods and Beverages			
Food	**Serving Size**	**Food**	**Serving Size**
5 Percent		Pork chop, grilled	3 ounces
Cashews	1 ounce	Salmon	3 ounces
Crab, cooked	3 ounces	**10 Percent**	
Kidney beans, boiled	⅓ cup	Haddock	3 ounces

RECOMMENDATIONS

When it comes to nutrition, there's a lot of important information to remember—so it helps to have what you need to know right at your fingertips. The most critical facts about selenium are summarized below.

What is the Optimal Daily Allowance of selenium?
The ODA of selenium for men and women is 200 micrograms.

What circumstances might affect the amount of selenium you need to take in each day?
Some lifestyle or health factors can affect the amount of selenium you consume or decrease the amount that your body is able to absorb and use. You'll have to be particularly conscientious about taking in the ODA of selenium if you are under physical or emotional stress; if you are vitamin E deficient; or if you are pregnant or breast-feeding.

Is it possible to consume the optimal amount of selenium through diet alone?
Surveys have shown that American men and women typically take in at least the RDA of selenium, but fall short of reaching the ODA. This may be due, in part, to the low selenium content of the soils in certain areas of the country.

Chapter 23

Other Important Minerals

The previous chapters in Part Three described some of the most important health-promoting minerals. Calcium, magnesium, zinc, iron, and selenium are necessary components of human nutrition that activate and control many physiological processes, from building strong, healthy bones to enhancing the immune system to preventing cancer. But the story doesn't end there.

Every cell in the body needs an array of mineral elements for its functioning and integrity, and survival depends on much more than the five minerals listed above. In fact, as nutritional science has become more sophisticated, researchers have found that there are actually seventeen essential minerals. Essential, as it is used here, means that the body cannot manufacture these nutrients, so they need to be taken in through diet.

All of the essential minerals were listed at the beginning of this book, in Chapter 1. As you may recall, some of these nutrients fall into the category of macro minerals, which are the major elements found in the human body. These include calcium and magnesium, as well as phosphorus, potassium, chloride, sodium, and sulfur. The rest of the minerals are called micro minerals, which are needed by the body in minute quantities. Zinc, selenium, and iron are considered to be micro minerals, as are chromium, cobalt, copper, fluoride, iodine, manganese, and molybdenum.

In this chapter, we'll briefly review some of the additional essential minerals and their uses in the body.

CHLORIDE

As you learned in Chapter 1, chloride is an electrolyte—a mineral salt that conducts the electrical energy needed to keep the body functioning. Along with other electrolytes, such as sodium and potassium, chloride helps move fluids into and out of the body's cells, ensuring that proper fluid balance is maintained in the body.

Chloride is a component of hydrochloric acid, the acid that breaks down food in the stomach. Hydrochloric acid aids the absorption of nutrients into the bloodstream and, as such, is necessary to maintain the body's internal balance, or homeostasis.

Finally, chloride is also an important factor in the transmission of nerve impulses.

Deficiency Symptoms

Chloride is found in many foods and can be obtained through a balanced diet. Therefore, deficiencies of this mineral are uncommon under normal circumstances. When chloride deficiency does develop, it usually occurs as the result of a strict salt-restricted diet, or following a severe and prolonged bout of vomiting and/or diarrhea.

Toxicity Symptoms

High intakes of chloride may cause vomiting. High blood pressure may also result from excessive chloride intake.

Optimal Daily Allowance

There is no RDA for chloride. The Optimal Daily Allowance ranges from 750 to 3,600 milligrams.

Few people need to take chloride supplements because deficiency is rare. When doctors recommend supplemental chloride, it is usually in the form of potassium chloride, a salt substitute.

Food Sources

Chloride is a primary component of table salt (sodium chloride). Salt and foods that contain salt are the principal dietary sources of chloride.

CHROMIUM

Chromium supports the activity of the hormone insulin, which helps glucose—or blood sugar—move into the body's cells. Glucose is the fuel that our cells "burn" for energy. Because it is involved in the metabolism of glucose, chromium is needed for energy. This mineral also assists the breakdown of carbohydrates and fats in the body.

Health Benefits

Chromium helps the body use insulin more efficienctly, and therefore plays a part in maintaining stable blood sugar levels. As such, the mineral may be helpful to people who have a decreased sensitivity to insulin. Some research has shown that individuals with type 2 non-insulin-dependent diabetes may benefit from chromium supplements.

In 1992, a Chinese study on the effects of chromium supplementation in people with type 2 diabetes was reported in the *Journal of the American College of Nutrition.* The participants—all of whom had type 2 diabetes—were divided into three groups of sixty people each. For four months, one group took a placebo with no active ingredients; a second group took 100 micrograms of chromium picolinate twice a day; and the third group took 500 micrograms of chromium picolinate twice a day. The group taking twice daily doses of 500 micrograms showed highly significant improvements in what the researchers called the "glucose/insulin system." Specifically, improvements were seen in the body's use of insulin, reflected in the patients' overall sensitivity to insulin. The group taking 100 micrograms of chromium picolinate showed a smaller degree of improvement or no significant improvement.

Some studies have shown that certain types of chromium supplements (for example, chromium-rich brewer's yeast) may decrease total cholesterol levels and increase "good" high-density lipoprotein (HDL) cholesterol. Research in this area has been very limited, however. A 1982 study published in the *Journal of the American College of Nutrition* involved twenty-seven adults, some of whom had normal cholesterol levels, and some of whom had high cholesterol levels. All of the participants took a daily 20-gram dose of chromium-rich brewer's yeast. The results showed that after eight weeks, both groups experienced significant decreases in total cholesterol (24 to 26 mg/dl) and increases in HDL cholesterol (5 to 6 mg/dl).

Chromium picolinate has been promoted as an aid for weight reduction and as a builder of muscle mass. In a German study conducted in 1997, researchers examined the effects of chromium picolinate on obesity in nondiabetic individuals, all around forty-five years of age. One group of participants took 200 micrograms a day of chromium picolinate, while the other group took a placebo. After twenty-six weeks, those participants taking the mineral showed significant increases in lean body mass and decreases in weight, compared with the placebo group.

Deficiency Symptoms

When chromium intake is inadequate, the body may use insulin less efficiently, which can result in abnormal blood glucose levels. In fact, people who take in low levels of chromium sometimes are mistakenly diagnosed as having diabetes because of elevated blood sugar levels. Chromium deficiency may also cause elevated cholesterol and triglyceride levels.

Toxicity Symptoms

In 1999, researchers at the University of Alabama suggested that high doses of chromium picolinate may cause genetic mutations when combined with antioxidants like vitamin C. However, their conclusions have been widely criticized because they were based on laboratory experiments that were not representative of chromium use in humans. No other signs of chromium toxicity have been identified.

People with diabetes are cautioned to speak with a doctor before self-prescribing chromium supplements, since supplementation could affect their required dosage of diabetes medications, including insulin. Because some evidence suggests that high doses of chromium can interfere with the absorption of iron and zinc, people who take in large amounts of chromium may need to consume more of these two minerals.

Optimal Daily Allowance

Information about the body's need for chromium is limited, and no RDA has been set for this mineral. The Optimal Daily Allowance of chromium is 200 micrograms, based on studies that demonstrate the importance of the nutrient in processes like carbohydrate metabolism. Most people consume considerably less of this mineral in their diets, however, averaging only 30 micrograms a day. You may need to be especially careful to take in the ODA of chromium if you exercise strenuously or if you include lots of simple sugars in your diet.

Chromium supplements are available in various forms, including chromium picolinate and chromium polynicotinate. Ongoing research should help clarify the potential benefits of each of these types of supplements.

Food Sources

The best dietary sources of chromium include brewer's yeast, liver, meat, shellfish, chicken, cheese, legumes, whole grains, and molasses.

COBALT

Your body contains approximately 1 milligram of cobalt. This mineral is a component of vitamin B_{12}, or cobalamin. In fact, vitamin B_{12} has the most complex structure of all vitamins, with a single cobalt atom positioned at its center.

Currently, all of cobalt's functions in the body are not fully understood. However, the mineral seems to be necessary for the manufacture of red blood cells, as well as for healthy nervous system function.

Deficiency Symptoms

Cobalt deficiency typically goes hand-in-hand with vitamin B_{12} deficiency. Therefore, inadequate intake of cobalt may result in pernicious anemia (see page 141), and may also cause a number of negative changes in the nervous system.

Toxicity Symptoms

Cobalt toxicity is virtually unknown as a nutritional disorder. Individuals who have been exposed to toxic levels of cobalt in factories and other occupational settings have been known to experience injury to red blood cells and skin cells.

Optimal Daily Allowance

No RDA or ODA has been established for cobalt.

Food Sources

Cobalt is plentiful in foods that contain vitamin B_{12}, including meat, fish, and milk and other dairy products.

COPPER

Copper plays a crucial role in the synthesis of hemoglobin, the iron-carrying component of red blood cells. It is also part of several important enzymes, including those that are essential for the formation of nerves and bones, and for the manufacture of collagen, an essential protein component of connective tissue, bones, and skin.

Copper plays a role in maintaining the integrity of myelin, the fatty substance that is a constituent of the covering of some nerves; keeping the heart and arteries functioning properly; and promoting healthy immune system function. Additionally, copper is a component of a number of enzymes, including those that are involved in the formation of bone and the manufacture of collagen, a component of connective tissue, bone, cartilage, and skin.

Deficiency Symptoms

Copper deficiency is unusual, despite the fact that the richest sources of dietary copper—such as liver and oysters—are not common in the typical American diet. However, people who take high doses of zinc supplements for a month or more may develop copper deficiency, since zinc impairs the body's absorption of copper. Also, the regular use of antacids has been shown to be a risk factor for copper deficiency, because these products interfere with copper absorption.

When copper deficiency does develop, symptoms include retarded growth, bone abnormalities, nervous system disorders, and hair loss. Also, as copper levels decline, iron absorption is impaired, which may cause anemia. Poor absorption may result in reduced enzyme activity that interferes with nervous system function, leading to poor concentration and lack of coordination. Some evidence suggests that people who are deficient in copper are at greater risk of developing heart and circulatory problems, particularly if a deficiency of selenium is also present.

Toxicity Symptoms

Copper toxicity can occur, sometimes from only a single 10-milligram dose. Symptoms of toxicity include nausea and vomiting, abdominal pains, diarrhea, headache, dizziness, and a metallic taste in the mouth. However, toxicity is rare in individuals who consume a normal diet and do not take copper supplements.

Optimal Daily Allowance

An RDA has not been established for copper. The Optimal Daily Allowance ranges from 1.5 to 3 milligrams. Nutritional surveys have shown that the average American falls just short of reaching the lower end of the ODA range—a typical intake is 1.2 to 1.3 milligrams daily.

There are a variety of copper supplements available, including copper aspartate, copper picolinate, and copper citrate. None of these forms seems to provide advantages over the others.

Food Sources

The best sources of copper include liver, kidney, shellfish (particularly oysters), raisins, nuts, legumes, whole grains, peas, artichokes, and radishes. Cooking your foods in a copper pot will increase their copper levels.

FLUORIDE

Fluoride promotes strong, healthy teeth by hardening tooth enamel. Fluoride's strengthening effects are most potent when the mineral is consumed during the years when tooth enamel and the underlying dentin are being formed (from birth to age eleven). In adults, fluoride promotes the remineralization of the enamel.

Health Benefits

Some research suggests that fluoride may also help prevent osteoporosis; some older people have shown improved bone strength in response to adequate fluoride intake. There is also evidence that the mineral may preserve existing bone mass in individuals who already have osteoporosis. In a study published in *The New England Journal of Medicine* in 1982, researchers examined the effects of fluoride supplementation on osteoporosis in 165 postmenopausal women. The women were divided into three groups: One group took supplements of calcium, vitamin D, or both; a second group supplemented with fluoride plus calcium and/or vitamin D; and a third group did not take mineral supplements. Some members of each of the three groups also took estrogen supplements. The researchers then monitored the incidence of vertebral fractures in the participants. The results showed that fluoride supplements provided significant protection against fractures—the incidence of vertebral fractures was lowest in the women taking fluoride. In the group taking fluoride, estrogen, and calcium (with or without vitamin D), the fracture rate was less than one-third as high, compared with the group taking only estrogen and calcium (with or without vitamin D).

Deficiency Symptoms

Fluoride deficiency may increase the risk of tooth decay. Also, some research has shown that deficiency may contribute to bone loss (osteoporosis) in adults.

Toxicity Symptoms

Toxic levels of fluoride can lead to dental fluorosis, a condition in which the teeth become mottled and pitted. This is primarily a cosmetic concern, and doesn't actually injure the teeth. Fluoride levels in community water supplies are maintained at low levels that will not cause fluorosis.

While some people have expressed fears that fluoridating drinking water may trigger serious illnesses such as cancer, the levels needed to protect against tooth decay are considered to be safe. The American Dental Association and other organizations have endorsed fluoridation because it reduces the risk of cavities by about 70 percent.

At much higher intakes, fluoride can cause toxicity symptoms that include nausea and vomiting, diarrhea, and itching.

Optimal Daily Allowance

An RDA for fluoride has not been established. The Optimal Daily Allowance ranges from 1.5 to 4 milligrams.

According to the American Dental Association, fluoride supplements are recommended for children up to age thirteen who live in communities where the fluoride concentration of tap water is under 0.7 parts of fluoride per million parts of water. The National Research Council recommends that drinking water be fluoridated to a level of 1 part per billion.

Food Sources

Sources of fluoride include tea and milk. Fish provides amounts of this mineral as well, if the bones are eaten—such as with anchovies and sardines. The best source of this mineral is fluoridated drinking water, from the tap or from a bottle.

IODINE

Iodine is a key component of the thyroid hormone *thyroxin,* which regulates metabolism, energy production, and growth. Iodine must be included in the diet for the body to produce thyroxin. Approximately three-quarters of the body's iodine content is located in the thyroid gland, while the remainder is distributed throughout the body, mostly in the fluids that bathe body cells.

Deficiency Symptoms

Deficiency stimulates the thyroid gland in an attempt to make increased quantities of thyroxin. However, this stimulus is incapable of increasing the output of thyroxin when ample iodine is lacking. The end result is the enlargement of the thyroid gland, which may become visible as a lump known as a goiter. Early in the twentieth century, goiter was commonly seen in the United States; once iodine was added to table salt, the incidence of goiter decreased dramatically.

Toxicity Symptoms

Goiter can also be a sign of iodine overdose, since excess iodine can interfere with the production of thyroxin. This symptom of iodine toxicity is seen more frequently in parts of the world where iodine-rich seaweed is included in the diet, such as in Japan.

Optimal Daily Allowance

The Optimal Daily Allowance of iodine is 150 to 200 micrograms. One-half teaspoon of iodized salt provides 200 micrograms.

Food Sources

The best food sources of iodine come from the sea. Iodized salt, as well as vegetables grown in iodine-rich soil, are also excellent sources of this mineral.

MANGANESE

Manganese is a component of many enzymes that facilitate chemical reactions throughout the body, including protein, fat, and carbohydrate metabolism. This mineral is also important for the normal growth and repair of bones and connective tissue; proper nervous system function; and immune system stimulation.

Deficiency Symptoms

Manganese is widely available in plant foods, so deficiency is rare.

In fact, deficiency symptoms have not been identified in humans. Although excessive iron or calcium can interfere with the absorption of manganese, this does not appear to cause problems in the body.

Toxicity Symptoms

Extremely high consumption of manganese can cause nerve disorders, although this occurs very rarely.

Optimal Daily Allowance

No RDA has been established for manganese. The Optimal Daily Allowance ranges from 2 to 5 milligrams.

Food Sources

The best sources of manganese are whole-grain cereals and breads, legumes, nuts, and seeds. Some fruits and vegetables—including strawberries and kale—also contain manganese.

MOLYBDENUM

Although it is found only in minute quantities in the body, molybdenum is an essential mineral for the maintenance of good health. This mineral works in conjunction with vitamin B_2 (riboflavin) to incorporate iron into hemoglobin, and thereby facilitates the production of red blood cells. It also activates several enzymes that promote normal cell function, and is required in extremely small amounts for nitrogen metabolism.

Deficiency Symptoms

Symptoms of molybdenum deficiency have not been identified in humans.

Toxicity Symptoms

Excessive intake of molybdenum can cause joint pain and may

result in copper deficiency because copper competes with molybdenum for absorption. High intakes of molybdenum can also cause excessive uric acid formation, and may therefore worsen the symptoms of gout.

Optimal Daily Allowance

An RDA has not been established for molybdenum. The Optimal Daily Allowance is 75 to 250 micrograms.

Food Sources

Molybdenum is found in whole-grain breads and cereals, milk, liver, beans, legumes, and dark green leafy vegetables.

PHOSPHORUS

Phosphorus is second only to calcium as the most abundant mineral in the human body. It is found in all of the body's cells and there are about one and a half pounds of it in an average-sized person. Most of the body's phosphorus—about 85 percent—is contained in the bones and teeth.

First and foremost, phosphorus works with calcium to build strong, healthy bones and teeth. But this mineral also plays a part in numerous chemical reactions in the body. Phosphorus is involved in the metabolism of carbohydrates, fats, and proteins for energy, and it is needed for cell formation, protein synthesis, and muscle contraction. The body also uses this nutrient to form enzymes and to help regulate enzyme activity.

Deficiency Symptoms

Phosphorus is present in some amount in nearly all foods, so deficiency is rare. The long-term use of aluminum-containing antacids, however, may interfere with phosphorus absorption and cause a deficit. When phosphorus deficiency does develop in people who are seriously malnourished, symptoms include weakness, loss of appetite, and loss of bone mass.

Toxicity Symptoms

Excessive phosphorus intake can reduce the amount of calcium in the blood, which may result in bone loss.

Optimal Daily Allowance

The Optimal Daily Allowance of phosphorus ranges from 800 to 1,200 milligrams. This recommendation parallels the RDA, which is 800 milligrams for adults ages twenty-five and over, and 1,200 milligrams for adolescents and young adults through age twenty-four. Because phosphorus is abundant in the diet, supplementation is rarely needed.

Food Sources

Foods that are especially high in phosphorus include milk and other dairy products, beef, poultry, fish, and eggs. Legumes, nuts, and whole-grain cereals and breads are also good sources of this mineral. And carbonated soft drinks contain phosphorus in the form of phosphoric acid.

POTASSIUM

Potassium is an electrolyte that is needed to maintain proper fluid balance within all of the body's cells. This mineral promotes normal metabolism, and is essential to nerve-impulse transmission and muscle contraction. A growing body of evidence indicates that potassium may also be instrumental in lowering high blood pressure.

Health Benefits

A number of studies have shown that people with high potassium intakes tend to have lower blood pressure than people who take in smaller amounts of the mineral. Researchers at Johns Hopkins University combined the data from thirty-three separate studies evaluating the effects of potassium supplementation on blood pressure. This meta-analysis, involving a total of 2,609 patients, found that potassium supplementation reduced the mean systolic and diastolic blood pressure by 3.11 and 1.97 mm Hg, respectively. Although this is not a major difference, even this amount may contribute to reductions in the likelihood of heart disease and stroke.

This potential positive impact is well demonstrated by a study done at the Harvard School of Public Health, and published in the journal *Circulation* in 1998. For eight years, researchers monitored 43,738 men (ages forty to seventy-five) without cardiovascular disease or diabetes. Over this time period, 328 of the men had strokes. The researchers found that those with the highest potassium intake (4.3 grams per day) were 38 percent less likely to have had a stroke, compared with those with the lowest intake (2.4 grams per day).

The positive effects of potassium on hypertension appear to be particularly strong in people with high intakes of sodium. In 1997, an article in *JAMA (The Journal of the American Medical Association)* reported that "increased potassium intake should be considered as a recommendation for the prevention and treatment of hypertension, especially in those who are unable to reduce their intake of sodium."

In Osaka, Japan, researchers at the National Cardiovascular Center studied the effect of potassium supplements on mild to moderate hypertension in fifty-five men and women, ages thirty-six to seventy-seven. All were given potassium supplements for four weeks, and then were monitored for another four weeks, during which time they did not take supplements. A report of the study in the *American Journal of Hypertension* in 1998 noted that blood pressure levels were lower while the subjects were taking potassium by an average of about 3 to 4 mm Hg—a small but clinically significant difference.

Deficiency Symptoms

Potassium deficiency is uncommon. Generally, deficiency results from factors such as alcoholism, vomiting, diarrhea, kidney disease, or diabetic acidosis. The excessive use of diuretics may cause the excretion of abnormally high levels of potassium, resulting in deficiency. Also, because the mineral can be lost through sweat, heavy exertion in hot weather may cause potassium levels to dip too low.

Symptoms of potassium deficiency include nausea and vomiting; loss of appetite; irritability; confusion; muscle weakness, muscle spasms, and cramps; and, in extreme cases, heart failure. Deficiency can also weaken bones and may cause slowed growth.

Toxicity Symptoms

Excessive amounts of potassium are usually excreted in the urine, so toxicity is rarely reported. However, kidney disease and other disorders may disrupt this balance and cause symptoms of toxicity. Very high blood levels of this mineral can cause muscle fatigue, irregular heartbeat, and possibly heart failure.

Optimal Daily Allowance

An RDA has not been established for potassium. The Optimal Daily Allowance ranges from 2,000 to 3,500 milligrams.

Individuals who are on very-low-calorie diets may need to take potassium supplements because they may not take in adequate amounts of the mineral from dietary sources. Supplementation may also be recommended for people who regularly use diuretics.

Food Sources

Milk, meats, poultry, and fish are all high in potassium. Legumes, fruits, vegetables, and whole grains are good sources of the mineral, as well.

SODIUM

Sodium is an electrolyte that helps maintain the volume and balance of all the fluids outside the body's cells, such as blood. This nutrient is important for muscle contraction and nerve-impulse transmission, and also helps to control cell permeability for easy exchange of substances across cell walls.

Deficiency Symptoms

Sodium must be consumed in the diet, since the body does not manufacture or store it. Deficiencies are unusual, and generally result from fasting, bouts of vomiting and/or diarrhea, excessive sweating, long-term diuretic use, or an overly strict low-sodium diet.

Symptoms of sodium deficiency include headaches, muscle cramps, muscle weakness, and loss of appetite.

Toxicity Symptoms

When sodium intake is excessive, fluid balance in the body can be disrupted and may cause symptoms of toxicity. These symptoms include hypertension and edema (swelling due to water retention).

Some people are considered to be "sodium sensitive"—their blood pressure climbs in response to sodium intake. This, in turn, increases their risk of developing heart disease, having a stroke, or suffering from kidney failure. There appears to be a hereditary component to sodium sensitivity; however, a decrease in sodium intake can lower blood pressure in these individuals.

In 1991, researchers at the Medical College of St. Bartholomew's Hospital in London reported on their analysis of seventy-eight existing studies on the effects of dietary salt and sodium reduction on blood pressure. The researchers found consistent decreases in blood pressure corresponding with decreases in sodium intake. For example, in individuals fifty to fifty-nine years old, reducing sodium intake by about 3 grams of table salt per day reduced systolic blood pressure readings by an average of 5 mm Hg, and 7 mm Hg in people with high blood pressure. Based on these results, the researchers estimated that if more people reduced sodium intake in this manner, the incidence of heart disease would be reduced by 15 percent, and stroke by 26 percent.

Optimal Daily Allowance

There is no RDA for sodium. The Senate Select Committee on Nutrition and Human Needs advises limiting sodium intake to no more than 2,000 milligrams daily (the equivalent of one teaspoon of salt), but most Americans consume much greater amounts.

The Optimal Daily Allowance of sodium ranges from 500 to 2,400 milligrams. In most industrialized countries, however, the daily intake of sodium is much greater, often averaging 5,000 to 7,500 milligrams.

Sodium is lost from the body as water is excreted through sweating. For this reason, people who exercise strenuously in hot weather may need to take in more of the mineral, approaching the higher end of the ODA range.

Food Sources

Common table salt is the main dietary source of sodium. Just one "pinch" of salt contains 267 milligrams of the mineral. Sodium is also present in moderate amounts in milk, meat, eggs, and certain vegetables, such as carrots, beets, spinach, and other leafy greens.

Nowadays, sodium is often an ingredient in many of the processed foods found on supermarket shelves and in fast-food restaurants. Pretzels and potato chips are the most obvious sources, but people are often surprised to learn that many soups and canned vegetables also contain added sodium. If you are trying to reduce your sodium intake, be sure to read nutrition labels carefully, since some products contain remarkably large amounts. You can also choose low-salt alternatives to the foods you enjoy.

SULFUR

Sulfur is found in all body tissues, making up about 0.25 percent of body weight. This mineral is part of the chemical structure of several amino acids, such as cysteine and methionine, and is needed for the synthesis of collagen, a component of connective tissue, bone, cartilage, and skin. Sulfur also helps to form keratin, which is required for healthy, strong hair and nails. Additionally, this mineral is a component of the hormone insulin—which helps glucose move into the body's cells—and of thiamin.

Deficiency Symptoms

Theoretically, sulfur deficiency could be asociated with a low-protein diet. Deficiency is extremely rare, however. In fact, symptoms have not been definitively identified in humans.

Toxicity Symptoms

Toxicity symptoms have not been reported with sulfur intake, since excess sulfur is excreted in the urine.

Optimal Daily Allowance

Neither an RDA nor an ODA has been established for sulfur.

Food Sources

Meat, fish, beans, dairy products, and eggs are high-protein foods that are good sources of sulfur.

VANADIUM

Although vanadium is an essential trace mineral, scientists knew little about its roles in the human body until recently. While the extent of its actions in the body has still not been completely defined, we do know that this mineral is needed for the formation of bones and teeth. It is also involved in cellular metabolism, human growth and development, and reproduction.

Health Benefits

Vanadium mimics the activity of insulin by promoting the transport of blood glucose into the body's cells, where it is used for energy. As such, the mineral may have benefits for some people with diabetes—especially individuals whose blood sugar levels are elevated because of *insulin resistance.* In people with this condition, body cells do not respond properly to insulin, so the pancreas must secrete more of the hormone to move glucose into the cells.

In a 1995 report printed in the *Journal of Endocrinology and Metabolism,* researchers announced the results of their study on the effects of vanadium supplements in people with diabetes. The researchers revealed that supplementation with the mineral resulted in improvements in glucose metabolism, insulin sensitivity, and blood cholesterol levels.

Vanadium may also offer benefits for individuals who have

mild degrees of insulin resistance associated with obesity. In these people, the mineral may facilitate the conversion of carbohydrates into a form of energy the body can use. This prevents excess carbohydrates from being stored as fat, and may be helpful in weight management.

Deficiency Symptoms

Only a small percentage of dietary vanadium is actually absorbed by the body—most is excreted in the urine. Animal studies have suggested that vanadium deficiency can retard normal growth and contribute to bone deformities, but deficiency symptoms in humans have not been reported.

Toxicity Symptoms

Vanadium toxicity rarely develops. When it does occur, symptoms such as diarrhea and cramping may result.

Optimal Daily Allowance

Neither an RDA nor an ODA has been established for vanadium. Studies have shown that Americans consume 10 to 100 milligrams of this mineral in their diets.

Food Sources

Food sources of vanadium include radishes, dill, whole grains, shellfish, mushrooms, and oats.

Part Four

The Herbs

Chapter 24

Black Cohosh

Black cohosh is the common name for *Cimicifuga racemosa*, a member of the buttercup family that grows in the woodlands of Eastern North America. Each plant bears a long stem that divides into several branches covered with small white flowers. The black root contains the active ingredients believed to be responsible for its medicinal benefits.

Traditionally, black cohosh has been used to relieve the discomforts of premenstrual syndrome (PMS), as well as menopausal symptoms such as hot flashes.

ACTIVE CONSTITUENTS

Black cohosh contains a variety of plant chemicals, including isoflavones, triterpene glycosides, isoferulic acid, oleic acid, palmitic acid, pantothenic acid, and phosphorus. Of these substances, much attention has focused on the *isoflavones,* which are chemically similar to the estrogens made by the body, although the plant chemicals are less potent. In particular, researchers have studied the effects of *formononetin,* an isoflavone present in black cohosh that binds to estrogen receptor sites in the body. Some researchers believe that formononetin is at least partly responsible for the herb's effectiveness in relieving menstrual and menopausal discomfort.

Some research has suggested that black cohosh relieves hot flashes by suppressing the release of *luteinizing hormone* (LH), a hormone secreted by the pituitary gland. When estrogen levels are

The History of Black Cohosh

For centuries, Native Americans have used black cohosh for a number of medical conditions, including infertility, irregular menstrual periods, sore throats, and rattlesnake bites. They boiled the root in water and then drank the decoction to treat their ailments.

In the nineteenth century, some physicians believed that black cohosh had anti-inflammatory properties, and recommended the herb to their patients to alleviate symptoms of arthritis. Black cohosh was also prescribed to relieve the pain of childbirth, and to treat menstrual irregularities and insomnia.

In the 1950s, serious research into black cohosh began, encouraged by doctors looking for a safe and effective treatment of symptoms associated with menopause. The positive findings of many of these studies has stimulated an interest in the herb, and today its use is becoming more widespread.

very low or absent (as they are after menopause) the pituitary gland releases bursts of LH in an attempt to stimulate the production of more estrogen by the ovaries. This is what triggers the hot flashes associated with menopause.

HEALTH BENEFITS

Germany's Commission E has approved the use of black cohosh root for premenstrual syndrome, menstrual pain, and symptoms associated with menopause. Several research studies support the use of black cohosh for these discomforts.

A study at the University of Gottingen in Germany evaluated the effects of black cohosh on the production of luteinizing hormone (LH) in 110 menopausal women. The participants received treatment with the herb for eight weeks. Researchers reported that the herb significantly reduced LH levels, with a corresponding decline in hot flashes.

Another German study, published in 1988, evaluated sixty women under forty years of age who had undergone hysterectomies; all subjects had at least one intact ovary, but still reported menopausal-like symptoms. The women were treated with either black cohosh extract or one of three conventional estrogen replacement therapies. Levels of LH were reduced in all treatment groups. Black cohosh produced comparable results to the traditional estrogen therapies.

In a multicenter study, published in the journal *Gyne* in 1982, investigators examined the effects of black cohosh extract on more than 600 menopausal women. Following eight weeks of treatment with the herb, 80 percent of the women reported improvement of menopausal symptoms such as hot flashes.

RECOMMENDED DOSAGE

Black cohosh is available in a variety of forms, including dried and fluid extracts, dried root in capsules, and tinctures. A daily dose of 40 milligrams of root extract standardized to contain 2.5-percent deoxyactein is typically recommended.

CONSIDERATIONS FOR USE

Black cohosh should not be used by pregnant women because of its estrogen-like properties. Also, women who are breast-feeding should not take the herb, since little information exists about its effects on lactation and its safety for children who are nursing. Germany's Commission E cautions that the herb should not be taken for more than six months because long-term studies of its effect on female hormones have not been conducted. The findings of studies that are now underway could change this recommendation, however.

Except for occasional stomach upset, side effects are rare when black cohosh is used at recommended doses. In very high doses, the herb can cause dizziness, vomiting, and a decrease in blood pressure.

Chapter 25

Cranberry

Vaccinium macrocarpon is the scientific name for the American cranberry, which is one of only three fruits native to North America. The cranberry plant is a small evergreen shrub that thrives in many different areas on the continent. Commercially, the plant is cultivated in Massachusetts and Wisconsin, as well as Eastern and Central Canada.

Cranberry juice is most often used in an attempt to treat urinary tract infections (UTIs). These infections are a common problem among women, although men may become more susceptible to infection with increasing age. UTIs occur when bacteria that are normally present in the intestine are introduced into the urinary tract and bladder.

ACTIVE CONSTITUENTS

At one time, it was believed that cranberries or cranberry juice could acidify the urine, thereby inhibiting the growth of bacteria and preventing urinary tract infections. However, more recent research suggests that cranberry prohibits *Escherichia coli*—the bacteria responsible for most UTIs—from adhering to the inner lining of the urinary tract. A study published in *The New England Journal of Medicine* in 1998 reported that chemical compounds called proanthocyanidins prevent bacteria from adhering to the wall of the urinary tract.

HEALTH BENEFITS

The effects of cranberry juice on urinary tract infections have been studied since the 1920s, but credible research remains rather limited. In 1994, researchers at Harvard Medical School reported the results of the first large-scale, placebo-controlled trial that demonstrated the ability of cranberry juice to prevent UTIs. This six-month-long trial involved 153 elderly women, divided into two groups: One group of women drank 300 milliliters per day of cranberry juice; the other consumed a cranberry-free placebo drink with the same color and taste, but with no active ingredients. The women were evaluated monthly for the presence of bacteria and white blood cells in their urine. The results—published in *JAMA (The Journal of the American Medical Association)*—revealed that participants who drank cranberry juice were 58 percent less likely to show evidence of asymptomatic urinary tract infections than those in the control group.

Note: Cranberries, cranberry juice, and cranberry extract are not acceptable alternatives to antibiotics when a urinary tract infection is present. Anyone who develops symptoms of a urinary tract infection should consult a physician for an accurate diagnosis and appropriate treatment.

RECOMMENDED DOSAGE

Although the optimal dose of cranberry has not been established, many health-care experts advise drinking 16 ounces of cranberry juice every day to prevent urinary tract infections. Also, concentrated cranberry juice extract is available in capsule form; the recommended dose is 300 to 400 milligrams taken twice daily.

CONSIDERATIONS FOR USE

No serious side effects have been reported with the use of cranberry juice or cranberry extract. Taking very large amounts may cause diarrhea in some individuals. Bear in mind that drinking a lot of cranberry juice can cause a significant increase in your calorie intake.

Chapter 26

Echinacea

Echinacea (pronounced eck-uh-*nay*-sha) is one of the most popular medicinal herbs available in the United States and Europe. The herb is used primarily as an immune system booster by people who want to increase their resistance to colds and other minor viral illnesses.

The echinacea plant is a member of the *Compositae* family, which also includes daisies, marigolds, and dandelions. It is indigenous to North America and grows wild throughout the United States, reaching a height of as much as three feet. The plant is also a favorite of gardeners because of its single purple flower with petals radiating outward from a cone-shaped center.

Although there are nine different species of echinacea, only three have been well studied and are used for medicinal purposes: *Echinacea angustifolia* (narrow-leafed coneflower), *Echinacea purpurea* (purple coneflower), and *Echinacea pallida* (pale coneflower). The roots and leaves of these plants are used for the healthful benefits they provide.

ACTIVE CONSTITUENTS

Echinacea contains a wide variety of natural chemicals that work together to stimulate the immune system, including polysaccharides, flavonoids, caffeic acid derivatives, polyacetylenes, alkylamides, and essential oils. The herb promotes a process called *phagocytosis*, in which white blood cells engulf infectious organisms, such as bacteria, viruses, and fungi. It also triggers an

---

The History of Echinacea

Native Americans used echinacea centuries ago. They applied it to wounds, used it as a mouthwash for toothaches, and drank echinacea tea to combat colds and arthritis.

In the latter part of the nineteenth century, physicians began recommending echinacea for colds, coughs, and sore throats. As word of its effectiveness spread, echinacea became a favorite of European healers as well. In the United States, the herb remained popular as an infection-fighter into the 1920s. There were even unsubstantiated claims that it was effective for everything from snake bites to migraines, and eczema to cancer.

With the development of antibiotics, interest in herbal remedies waned, although echinacea was listed until 1950 in the *National Formulary*, a pharmacists' reference book. In recent years, echinacea has made an impressive comeback, due in part to a consumer-driven trend toward natural medicine that has fueled an interest in herbal remedies in general. The herb's popularity has also been helped by positive statements about it in Germany's Commission E report and by some positive results from a number of recent studies.

---

increase in the release of infection-fighting proteins known as interferons.

HEALTH BENEFITS

Several hundred scientific studies and reports have been published about echinacea and its benefits. Enough credible evidence has accumulated to convince Germany's Federal Health Agency (that country's equivalent of the U.S. Food and Drug Administration) to formally approve echinacea as a supportive or auxiliary treatment for the common cold, influenza, urinary tract infections, and hard-to-heal superficial wounds.

The most reliable studies of echinacea have been conducted in Germany. Most of this research has evaluated the effectiveness of liquid preparations obtained from the flowering part of the echinacea plant. For example, in research published in 1992, nearly 200 people with the flu, ranging in age from eighteen to sixty years old, took high doses of *Echinacea purpurea* extract, and were compared with a group taking a placebo with no active ingredients. The participants who took the equivalent of four droppersful of echinacea had a 75 percent greater decrease in flu symptoms, such as sore throat and stuffy nose, within three to four days. However, individuals taking a lower dose did no better than the placebo group.

A German study of echinacea's effects on the common cold, published in 1992, involved more than 100 people, all of whom had three or more colds during the previous winter. One group took 2 to 4 milliliters of *Echinacea purpurea* twice a day for eight weeks; the other group took a placebo. The results showed that echinacea did, in fact, decrease the participants' chances of developing a cold—35 percent in the echinacea group stayed healthy, compared with 26 percent in the placebo group. Supplementation with echinacea also increased the time between infections. Individuals in the echinacea group remained healthy for approximately forty days, compared with twenty-five days for individuals in the placebo group. When participants taking echinacea did catch colds, their symptoms were less severe and of shorter duration.

In 1998, German researchers reported a study of nearly 300 people who took fifty drops twice daily of herbal root extracts of *Echinacea purpurea* or *Echinacea angustifolia*, or a placebo. After twelve weeks of supplementation, 32 percent and 29 percent of the individuals taking *E. purpurea* and *E. angustifolia*, respectively, had caught at least one cold. However, these results were not statistically better than those seen in the placebo group; after twelve weeks, 37 percent of the people taking the placebo developed colds. Nevertheless, participants in both of the echinacea groups subjectively *believed* that they benefited more than individuals taking the placebo. The researchers also reported a trend towards a 10 to 20 percent reduction in cold risk, which they said might have been more clearly demonstrated in a larger study with more patients.

Other investigators have reported other benefits of echinacea, but more research needs to be done to substantiate these claims. While there are individual case reports of echinacea helping people with disorders such as psoriasis, eczema, candidiasis, rheumatoid arthritis, headaches, and urinary tract infections, there is insufficient scientific evidence at this time to recommend echinacea for these purposes.

RECOMMENDED DOSAGE

Echinacea is available in a number of forms, including capsules, tablets, liquid extracts, and teas. For products made from echinacea roots, a typical recommended dose in Germany is 900 milligrams per day, divided into two to three equal doses. Alcohol tinctures of *Echinacea purpurea* are usually taken in doses of thirty to sixty drops, three times a day. For colds, you can try drinking echinacea tea several times throughout the day. Follow the directions on the label of the particular product you choose.

Most health-care professionals trained in herbal medicine recommend taking echinacea at the first sign of a cold or flu, and continuing treatment for ten to fourteen days. According to Germany's Commission E, echinacea should not be taken for more than eight weeks at a time, since its effectiveness will decrease over time. Thus, echinacea should not be used prophylactically in hopes of keeping colds and the flu at bay.

CONSIDERATIONS FOR USE

According to Germany's Commission E, there are no known side effects when echinacea is taken by mouth or used as an ointment. The U.S. Food and Drug Administration has received a small number of reports of adverse effects associated with the herb, including abdominal distress; however, the FDA has not been able to confirm that echinacea was actually responsible for these symptoms. In animal studies, no side effects have been linked to the herb, even when it was taken in very high doses.

Because echinacea can affect the immune system, people with autoimmune disorders, such as rheumatoid arthritis, lupus, and multiple sclerosis, should not use this herb. Individuals with progressive chronic illnesses are typically not considered good candidates for echinacea therapy; thus, individuals with HIV infection, diabetes, and tuberculosis may be advised against supplementing with the herb.

You should not use echinacea if you are allergic to plants related to echinacea, including sunflowers, daisies, marigolds, and chrysanthemums.

Chapter 27

Evening Primrose

The evening primrose plant—known in the scientific community as *Oenothera biennis*—is indigenous to North America, but was introduced in Europe and parts of Asia as early as the seventeenth century. Evening primrose is a hardy, drought-tolerant plant that grows well in a variety of environments, and is even known to thrive in fallow lands and sandy soils. The plant's large, yellow flowers usually open between six and seven o'clock in the evening—hence the name, evening primrose. (This herb also goes by other names, including night-willow herb, fever plant, and sun drop.) The plant produces small but fertile seeds, from which the oil is extracted. Evening primrose oil is most often used to treat conditions such as atopic eczema, premenstrual syndrome (PMS), and diabetic neuropathy, although more research is needed in all of these areas.

ACTIVE CONSTITUENTS

Evening primrose oil, extracted from the seeds of the plant, is an excellent source of *essential fatty acids* (EFAs), which are necessary for health and cannot be manufactured by the body. EFAs are essential to proper brain and nervous system function; help maintain the structure and function of cell membranes; and promote healthy skin, hair, and nails. They have also been found to reduce blood cholesterol.

The oil from the evening primrose seeds contains ingredients called *linoleic acid* and *gamma-linolenic acid* (GLA), which are believed to be key ingredients for the therapeutic benefits associated with this herb. In particular, GLA is a precursor to *prostaglandins* (PGE1), hormone-like substances that help regulate the central nervous system and the immune system, and perform other physiological functions. Prostaglandins also appear to have anti-inflammatory properties.

HEALTH BENEFITS

Evening primrose oil (EPO) is often used to relieve the symptoms of atopic eczema, a chronic condition that causes dry, itchy, and inflamed skin, but there is conflicting evidence about its effectiveness. In a double-blind study reported in 1987 in the *British Journal of Dermatology*, Finnish researchers compared evening primrose oil (taken orally) to a placebo in twenty-five patients with atopic eczema. After twelve weeks, the researchers detected a significantly greater improvement in the group taking the herb than in the group taking the placebo, including a reduction in the severity of their skin inflammation and the percentage of their body surface affected by the eczema, as well as a decrease in dryness and itchiness. However, other studies have failed to produce these positive results with EPO.

Evening primrose oil has also been used to treat symptoms of premenstrual syndrome (PMS), although studies in this area have produced conflicting results. In 1985, researchers at Oulu University Hospital in Finland reported that 3 grams of evening primrose oil per day could ease symptoms such as breast tenderness and depression in women with PMS. Subsequently, investigators at the University of Queensland in Australia compared evening primrose oil with placebo treatments in thirty-eight women with PMS symptoms, and reported no differences in the two groups—in fact, both groups improved slightly. In 1996, researchers at Queen's University of Belfast's School of Pharmacy reviewed all of the studies that had been conducted on the effect of evening primrose oil in the treatment of PMS and concluded that the herb "is of little value in the management of premenstrual syndrome."

The use of evening primrose oil has also been studied in people with diabetic neuropathy. This condition is characterized by numbness, burning, and tingling—usually in the feet—caused by an insufficient supply of blood to the nerves. In a study published in *Diabetes Care* in 1993, researchers at Guy's Hospital and other centers in the United Kingdom evaluated the effects when patients with mild diabetic neuropathy took GLA (found in evening prim- rose) at a dose of 480 milligrams per day. Over a one-year period, they found that in measurements of sixteen different parameters, the course of the condition improved in those using GLA. For example, their muscle strength and overall sensations became bet- ter, compared with a control group not taking GLA.

RECOMMENDED DOSAGE

The optimal dose of evening primrose oil has not been clearly defined, although the usual recommended dose is 3 to 6 grams of EPO per day.

CONSIDERATIONS FOR USE

No side effects have been identified with the use of evening prim- rose oil taken at the recommended dosage levels.

Chapter 28

Feverfew

Feverfew, or *Tanacetum parthenium*, is a perennial that thrives throughout North America, Europe, and Australia. The plant grows to about two or three feet in height, with a slender trunk branching out into several stems that bear strongly aromatic yellow-green leaves. From mid-summer to early fall, the feverfew plant blooms with abundant daisy-like flowers, which have white petals radiating outward from their nearly flat yellow centers. The dried flowers and leaves of the herb are most often used in medicinal preparations.

The name feverfew is derived from the Latin word *febrifugia*, meaning "chase away fevers," and the herb has a long history of use for this purpose in traditional and folk medicine. However, scientific investigation of the active constituents of this herb have not revealed any temperature-lowering properties. Instead, there is evidence indicating that feverfew can help reduce the frequency and severity of migraine headaches.

ACTIVE CONSTITUENTS

Parthenolide appears to be the primary active constituent of feverfew. The compound prevents the release of serotonin, a neurotransmitter that—among many other effects in the body—causes the blood vessels in the head to dilate. By blocking the release of serotonin, feverfew may prevent this dilation and the accompanying headaches.

The History of Feverfew

In the first century AD, the Greek physician Dioscorides wrote about the use of feverfew in the text *De Materia Medica;* he described it as an herb appropriate for "all hot inflammations." In the early twentieth century, feverfew was widely prescribed in England as an analgesic for the treatment of arthritis, but then its popularity waned. In the last two decades, the herb has enjoyed a resurgence in use, due in part to its approval by Canadian and British government agencies for migraine therapy.

HEALTH BENEFITS

A number of well-designed studies have confirmed a role for feverfew in the treatment of migraine headaches. One study conducted at University Hospital in Nottingham, England, and published in *The Lancet* in 1988, looked at the effects of feverfew on migraine headaches in seventy-two men and women. For four months, the participants took either 82 milligrams a day of dried feverfew leaves (containing 500 micrograms of parthenolide) in capsule form or a placebo, with no active ingredients. Then, each group was switched to the other treatment for the next four months. While taking feverfew, participants experienced a significant decline in migraine frequency and severity, as well as fewer headache-related vomiting episodes and visual disturbances. Interestingly, side effects actually occurred less frequently in the feverfew groups, compared with groups taking the placebo.

In 1985, the *British Medical Journal* published the results of a study looking at the benefits of feverfew in seventeen people with histories of migraine headaches. Nearly half of the participants took 50 milligrams a day of freeze-dried, powdered feverfew extract, while the rest of the participants took a placebo. The researchers found that individuals in the feverfew group experienced fewer migraines than those in the placebo group; when headaches did occur, they were milder and less incapacitating.

Researchers in Israel evaluated feverfew's ability to prevent future headaches or to minimize headache severity in fifty-seven migraine patients. The participants of the study took either 100 milligrams a day of feverfew or a placebo for a total of four months. The group supplementing with feverfew experienced a significant reduction in pain intensity, compared with the group taking the placebo. There was also a decline in symptoms that commonly accompany migraines—nausea, vomiting, and sensitivity to light and noise—in the feverfew group. In their article published in *Psychotherapy Research,* the researchers concluded that "feverfew appears to be the most practical way to block completely, to slow down, or to ease migraine and headaches as well as to prevent the side effects associated with the common drug practices."

Not all studies have reached such positive conclusions about feverfew, however. For instance, Dutch researchers discovered that feverfew did not reduce the incidence of migraines in the fifty people they studied. During the first four months of this study, participants took feverfew supplements containing 0.5 milligrams of parthenolide in capsule form as a daily prophylactic treatment for migraines. During a separate four-month cycle of the study, all of these individuals took a placebo every day. The outcome of this study, reported in 1996 in *Phytomedicine,* showed that patients suffered the same number of migraine headaches when they took feverfew as when they took the placebo.

Although some herbalists recommend feverfew as a treatment for rheumatoid arthritis (RA), the research conducted thus far has not supported its use for this particular condition. In a British study published in the *Annals of Rheumatic Diseases* in 1989, researchers concluded that feverfew does not help relieve the symptoms of rheumatoid arthritis. This study involved forty-one women with RA, who took either 70 to 86 milligrams a day of dried feverfew or a placebo. Over the course of six weeks, symptoms did not differ between the two groups. The researchers stated that there was "no apparent benefit from oral feverfew in rheumatoid arthritis."

RECOMMENDED DOSAGE

Fresh leaves of feverfew are available for medicinal purposes, and the herb can also be found in capsule form. The recommended dosage is 250 micrograms of parthenolide per day. Be aware that feverfew capsules can vary considerably in their content of active compounds, such as parthenolide, which are thought by many researchers to be responsible for the herb's benefits. For this reason, you should always choose products containing a standardized feverfew extract.

Feverfew works best in the prevention of migraine headaches, rather than as a pain reliever once a headache has already developed. Some people who abruptly stop taking the herb may experience rebound headaches.

CONSIDERATIONS FOR USE

Feverfew must not be taken by women who are pregnant or breast-feeding, and should not be given to children under two years of age. Because of reports that the herb can interact with some medications, such as aspirin and warfarin (Coumadin), it's important to seek the advice of a health-care practitioner before undertaking a treatment regimen.

Chewing feverfew leaves has been implicated in the development of mouth ulcers. Use of the herb may also cause dermatitis, an inflammation of the skin that produces scaling, flaking, and itching. Other side effects, such as stomach upset, can occur, but these effects are not common.

Chapter 29

Garlic

P eople all over the world use garlic to enhance the flavor of their meals, and it seems that Americans just can't get enough of it. About 250 million pounds of fresh garlic are consumed as food in the United States each year! This pungent herb, known in the scientific community as *Allium sativa*, is also one of the top-rated remedies in households around the world.

The garlic plant is a member of the family *Liliaceae*, and is a close relative of onion, chives, and leeks. Its stem grows to about two feet in height, ending in a cluster of pink, red, or white flowers. The base of the stem is expanded into a fat bulb, which contains six to twelve cloves, enclosed in a papery sheath. These cloves, when dried, are known for the distinctive flavor they impart to foods, and they have also been used for thousands of years for their medicinal properties.

Research has confirmed that taking garlic may lower cholesterol and blood pressure levels, although its effects are modest.

ACTIVE CONSTITUENTS

Garlic contains more than a dozen amino acids, which are the building blocks of proteins; several vitamins, including A, B_1, B_2, and C; a variety of minerals, including germanium, iron, magnesium, manganese, phosphorus, potassium, selenium, sulfur, and zinc; and thirty-three different sulfur compounds.

The principal active ingredient in garlic is the sulfur-containing compound *allicin*. Allicin is created from the sulfur compound

The History of Garlic

Garlic has a history of use as food and medicine that spans thousands of years. The dried herb was found among precious metals and jewels buried in the tombs of the Pharaoh Tutankhamen and, according to some inscriptions, the builders of the great pyramids consumed large amounts of garlic. The herb was also used thousands of years ago by the ancient Greeks and Romans, who valued it as a source of strength. In these civilizations, garlic was used to treat breathing problems, eliminate parasites, alleviate indigestion, and promote weight loss. Garlic was used liberally during the time of the early Chinese dynasties to treat snakebite, and to eliminate pinworms and fungal infections. In ancient India, the people celebrated a special festival devoted to garlic.

Throughout the centuries, people in many areas of the world developed their own ideas about how garlic can be used to ward off evil spirits, or to keep vampires and demons at bay. Although the ancient Greeks and Romans acknowledged garlic as having mystical powers, the notion that the herb has supernatural properties appeared to have been popularized largely because of the novel *Dracula*.

Only in the last few centuries has garlic undergone serious scientific scrutiny. In 1858, Louis Pasteur identified antibacterial properties in this plant. As recently as World War II, Russian soldiers turned to garlic cloves to treat infections when they ran out of antibiotics. Today, there's some evidence that garlic has beneficial effects on cholesterol levels and the cardiovascular system.

alliin, when the fresh garlic cloves are cut, crushed, or cooked. Allicin is not only responsible for garlic's pungent odor and flavor, but researchers believe that it is also one of the sources of the herb's health benefits. In laboratory studies, allicin has demonstrated antibacterial and antifungal activity against many common organisms.

Garlic may also provide some protection against cardiovascular disease because of its mild cholesterol-lowering properties, and because it stimulates fibrinolysis, the process by which blood clots are dissolved. A compound known as *ajoene,* isolated from garlic, appears to be responsible for this benefit.

HEALTH BENEFITS

Garlic has probably been studied more extensively than any other herb—more than 1,000 studies have been published on its possible medicinal benefits. Germany's Commission E has approved garlic as a dietetic approach for managing high blood cholesterol levels and preventing "age-dependent vascular changes" such as fatty deposits in the lining of the arteries.

To date, over thirty studies have been conducted to determine garlic's effects on blood cholesterol in humans. One study, carried out at Tulane University, involved forty-two men and women with high blood cholesterol levels. The participants were divided into two groups: One group took three 300-milligram capsules of powdered garlic extract daily—equivalent to one and a half cloves of garlic a day—while the other group took a placebo. After twelve weeks, the group taking the garlic experienced a 6 percent decline in total cholesterol and an 11 percent drop in their levels of "bad" low-density lipoprotein (LDL) cholesterol. In contrast, total cholesterol and LDL cholesterol levels decreased only one and three percent, respectively, in the individuals taking the placebo.

At New York Medical College, researchers combined data from five previously conducted studies of garlic's effects on cholesterol levels, involving a total of more than 400 people. They concluded that garlic supplements, in doses equivalent to one-half to one clove of garlic a day, lowered cholesterol levels by an average of nine percent.

As promising as the results of these and many more studies have been, some research has failed to find a link between garlic supplements and reduced cholesterol. One such study was conducted by German researchers, and involved twenty-five patients with high total cholesterol—240 to 348 mg/dl. Every day for three months, the participants took garlic oil preparations equaling 4 to 5 grams of fresh garlic cloves. This was followed by a one-month "wash-out" period, after which the participants took a placebo daily for another three months. The result? According to this study, published in *JAMA (The Journal of the American Medical Association)*, garlic oil supplements had no effect on cholesterol or triglyceride levels. It's important to note, however, that this study was criticized for its small size and because garlic oil is reported not to work as well as the powdered extract.

In a study of artery elasticity, which was published in the journal *Circulation* in 1996, German investigators reported that people who consumed about 500 milligrams of garlic supplements a day—equal to less than one clove—for an average of seven years had more flexible arteries than individuals who did not take the supplements. Another German study, published in the same journal in 1997, concluded that when healthy adults took 300 to 900 milligrams a day of powdered garlic preparations for two years or more, they had significantly reduced pulse wave velocity of the aorta, which indicates a reduced workload for the heart.

Several recent studies have found that stomach and colon cancer rates are much lower in regions of the world where garlic is a regular part of the diet. In 1989, a large study sponsored by the U.S. National Cancer Institute was conducted in the Shandong province of China, where the population has a high incidence of stomach cancer. Researchers compared the diets of 564 Chinese people with stomach cancer to the diets of 1,131 people who were cancer-free. Participants who had high dietary intakes of garlic and its relatives—onions, scallions, Chinese chives—had a 60 percent lower chance of developing stomach cancer, compared with individuals who did not consume garlic as a regular part of their diets.

However, research has not always produced positive results about garlic's benefits as an anticancer agent. A Dutch study involving 2,100 women concluded that the use of garlic supplements was not associated with a decreased risk of breast cancer. Another Dutch study, which involved 3,600 men, found that garlic supplements did not reduce the risk of lung cancer.

Many herbal experts believe that garlic is not as potent a cholesterol-lowering agent as some people need, and therefore should not be substituted for conventional medical therapy. For example, in people with blood cholesterol levels greater than 240 mg/dl, garlic is unlikely to drop cholesterol levels into the "desirable" zone. These people should consider more aggressive measures, such as cholesterol-lowering prescription drugs. For those with milder elevations in their cholesterol levels, a trial with garlic and/or other nutritional supplements may be appropriate. Traditional medical therapy should be considered, however, if a prompt and adequate response is not achieved.

RECOMMENDED DOSAGE

Germany's Commission E recommends an average daily dose of 4 grams of fresh garlic or its equivalent. Taking one to two fresh garlic cloves a day will be enough to reap all of the healthful benefits that the herb provides. For those who don't want to include fresh garlic in their daily diet, there are many different types of garlic supplements available, including dried garlic tablets and deodorized garlic, which come in capsule or tablet form. Garlic oil is also available, but a recent study of this preparation showed that it does not have the same cholesterol-lowering properties as dried garlic.

CONSIDERATIONS FOR USE

Garlic has an anticoagulant effect on blood. Thus, large amounts should not be consumed by people who are taking anticoagulant (blood-thinning) medications, including aspirin and warfarin (Coumadin). If you are taking these medications, discuss the advisability of consuming garlic with your physician.

For many people, the most troubling side effect of this herb is "garlic breath." Eating some parsley or lettuce or chewing a few seeds of fennel after consuming garlic may help to neutralize the odor. If you're worried about the effect that garlic odor might have on your social life, the best way to take the herb is in supplement form.

Garlic is exceptionally safe, and few adverse effects have been reported by people who consume large amounts of the herb daily in food or supplement form. Some experience heartburn or mild digestive discomfort after consuming garlic, but this effect usually does not last for long.

Chapter 30

Ginger

Most people think of ginger as a flavorful spice, but this pungent herb has a long history of use for its medicinal benefits. Dried ginger root has been used for thousands of years in Chinese and Ayurvedic medicine. In addition to its properties as a flavoring agent, ginger—known scientifically as *Zingiber officinale*—has been used for gastrointestinal ailments, including nausea, vomiting, motion sickness, gas, and stomach cramps. The parts of the plant used for therapeutic purposes are the rhizome (underground stem) and the root.

ACTIVE CONSTITUENTS

The oils of the ginger plant—including camphene, phellandrene, sesquiterpene, zingiberene, cineoloe, citral, and borneol—are largely responsible for its distinctive aroma and pungent taste, and perhaps even more. Animal studies have shown that a substance called *oleoresin*, which is contained in these oils, may improve the tone and activity of the gastrointestinal tract, and can counter tendencies toward nausea and vomiting.

HEALTH BENEFITS

Ginger's ability to improve digestion and relieve gastrointestinal distress has been demonstrated in many research studies. In Germany, Switzerland, and Australia, the use of ginger is approved for the prevention of motion sickness and the relief of dyspepsia, or indigestion.

In one early study, published in 1982, researchers administered 940 milligrams a day of either powdered ginger or Dramamine to more than thirty college students who had a history of motion sickness. Within thirty minutes after consuming the Dramamine or ginger, the participants were asked to sit on a rotating chair designed to induce motion sickness. The results, which were reported in *The Lancet,* showed that the ginger group lasted 57-percent longer on the chair before symptoms of motion sickness prompted them to ask for the experiment to stop.

At Louisiana State University Medical Center, researchers evaluated ginger's effects on motion sickness in twenty-eight volunteers. The participants took 500 to 1,000 milligrams of powdered ginger, 1,000 milligrams of fresh ginger root, or a medication called scopolamine, which is sometimes used to treat motion sickness, and then were asked to sit on a rotating chair designed to induce motion sickness. In an article published in *Pharmacology* in 1991, the investigators reported that, although powdered ginger did interfere with the increased rate of stomach contractions (tachygastria) associated with motion sickness, it did not significantly reduce the symptoms of motion sickness.

Some studies have also shown that ginger can prevent or reduce the nausea and vomiting of morning sickness. A study at the University of Copenhagen, published in 1991, found that 1 gram per day of powdered ginger root, taken for four days, was better than a placebo in easing or eliminating the symptoms of hyperemesis gravidarum in nineteen women. Hyperemesis gravidarum is a form of morning sickness that may be severe enough to require hospitalization.

A word of caution is in order: While some herbalists recommend the use of ginger to alleviate the symptoms of morning sickness, many others are cautious about recommending the use of *any* herb during pregnancy. Although there is no evidence that ginger can harm either the expectant mother or the fetus, Germany's Commission E advises against the use of this herb during pregnancy.

RECOMMENDED DOSAGE

Germany's Commission E recommends a daily dose of 2 to 4 grams of ginger a day for dyspepsia and the prevention of motion sickness. Ginger is available in capsules containing 250 to 500 milligrams of the powdered herb. A typical regimen is to take two capsules (0.5 to 1 gram) about thirty minutes before your ship or plane departs, and up to two additional capsules every four hours as needed.

To prepare ginger tea, simmer 1 ounce of fresh or one-half ounce of dried ginger root for 10 minutes in 1 pint of water. Add honey to sweeten the tea, if you wish.

CONSIDERATIONS FOR USE

No side effects have been reported when ginger is taken at the recommended doses.

People who have gallstones should consult with a health-care practitioner before self-administering ginger; this herb appears to increase the flow of bile into the intestine, which may aggravate the problem of gallstones.

Chapter 31

Ginkgo Biloba

Ginkgo biloba is an herbal extract from the leaves of the gink-go tree, the oldest living species of tree on the planet. The ginkgo tree is the only survivor of the *Ginkgoaceae* family and has a fossil history going back 200 million years. This tree is native to China, but now grows in many parts of the world, mostly in temperate climates. It is hardy enough to thrive in adverse conditions, including drought and pollution, and it is highly resistant to insects and parasites. Because of this, an individual ginkgo tree can survive for a thousand years!

While ginkgo has been used for over five thousand years in traditional Chinese medicine, it has become a popular herbal treatment in the United States relatively recently. These days, ginkgo extract is most often used to treat circulatory disorders and memory loss, and to sharpen cognitive abilities. In the past twenty years, European practitioners have been prescribing ginkgo for people with cognitive decline associated with aging. It has also been used for circulatory disorders such as intermittent claudication. In recent years, ginkgo has become one of the most widely used herbal remedies in the United States as well, and it continues to be the subject of increasing scientific scrutiny.

ACTIVE CONSTITUENTS

Ginkgo's active ingredients included bioflavonoids called *ginkgo flavone glycosides*, as well as terpene lactones. The flavone glyco-

The History of Ginkgo

One of the earliest records of ginkgo's use in Chinese medicine comes from the medical text *Pen T'sao Ching*, reportedly written by Emperor Shen Nung (2839–2698 BC). The Emperor, who is considered the first Chinese herbalist, found the most important use of ginkgo very early—he observed that ginkgo leaves appeared to enhance cognitive abilities. Chinese herbalists also used the leaves to relieve asthma and cough, and the seeds to aid digestion; however, modern scientific study has not proven the herb to possess these benefits.

Europeans first encountered the ginkgo tree in the early eighteenth century. They took it home to Europe, where it became popular as an ornamental tree, particularly in urban areas. Carolus Linnaeus, the great Swedish botanist, called the tree *Ginkgo biloba*, meaning "ginkgo with two lobes," because its leaves are divided in two by a notch. In 1784, soon after the American Revolution, the ginkgo tree was brought to North America.

sides function as antioxidants, neutralizing the toxic effects of free radicals, which some researchers believe may contribute to the brain cell injury in Alzheimer's disease.

Ginkgo also appears to improve blood flow within the brain, which may contribute to cognitive improvements.

HEALTH BENEFITS

Ginkgo has been singled out by Germany's Commission E as effective therapy for memory deficits and concentration problems associated with aging. It is also used to combat *tinnitus,* or ringing in the ears, and *claudication,* which refers to leg cramps that occur during walking—both fairly common conditions among older people. Plus, ginkgo may be sued to relieve dizziness and a more serious porblem known as *vertigo,* which is the sensation that one's surroundings are spinning..

Much of the excitement about ginkgo's ability to improve mild memory and concentration problems grew out of a study published in *JAMA (The Journal of the American Medical Association)* in 1997—the first large-scale American clinical trial of ginkgo. Investigators from several respected institutions, including the New York Institute for Medical Research and Harvard Medical School, evaluated 202 men and women with mild to moderately severe dementia caused by Alzheimer's disease and/or strokes. Half of these people were treated with 120 milligrams of ginkgo extract per day (in three 40-milligram pills); the other half received placebos.

Six months to a year later, 50 percent of those in the ginkgo group experienced improvements in memory, language, and reasoning; interestingly, similar improvements occurred in 29 percent of those taking placebos. About 37 percent of the people on ginkgo performed better at activities of daily living, compared with 23 percent of their placebo counterparts. (These activities included the ability to manage money, recognize familiar faces, and carry on a conversation.) The researchers concluded that the improvements related to the use of ginkgo extract "may be equivalent to a six-month delay in the progression of the disease."

Other studies have confirmed that ginkgo may have a positive effect on cognitive functioning. In 1998, investigators at Oregon Health Sciences University published a meta-analysis (combining the data from several studies) involving a total of 424 Alzheimer's patients who had been randomly assigned to receive either ginkgo or a placebo. After three to six months, those in the herb group scored 3 percent higher on tests for learning and memory, compared with those who took a placebo—a relatively small but statistically significant improvement.

Ginkgo may also be effective in treating certain circulatory conditions, such as intermittent claudication. The herb appears to improve circulation by dilating the blood vessels. Ginkgo has also been used by some practitioners for the treatment of Raynaud's phenomenon, a disorder in which the fingers and toes become unusually cool, pale, and painful when exposed to cold or during emotional distress; the pallor and coolness is caused by constriction of the arteries supplying blood to the extremities.

No scientific studies have shown that ginkgo can *prevent* dementia or Alzheimer's disease. Its primary benefits are for alleviation of symptoms in people with mild cognitive impairment.

RECOMMENDED DOSAGE

Ginkgo extracts are available in liquid, tablet, or capsule form. The usual recommended dose is 120 to 240 milligrams a day in two to three divided doses. Choose a standardized extract containing 24-percent ginkgo flavone glycosides and 6-percent terpene lactones. This is the preparation used in most studies of ginkgo. Be aware that it may be necessary to take ginkgo for six to eight weeks before improvements in memory become apparent.

CONSIDERATIONS FOR USE

Ginkgo may have anticoagulant properties; for that reason, some physicians advise against its use if you're already taking other blood-thinning medications such as warfarin (Coumadin) and aspirin. If you take these medications and you are interested in supplementing with ginkgo, make sure you get the go-ahead from your health-care practitioner first.

There are no serious side effects associated with the use of ginkgo. However, a very small percentage of users have reported mild reactions such as stomach upset, headaches, and allergic skin reactions.

Chapter 32

Ginseng

Ginseng is a unique herb that has been used for over 2,000 years in traditional Eastern medicine. Throughout the centuries, ginseng root has been highly valued for its tonic properties, recommended by herbalists to strengthen health and restore vitality. Now it has become quite popular in the West, as well, used mainly to combat stress and fatigue, and to give the immune system a boost. The herb has become so popular, in fact, that it is even added to candy, snack bars, and other foods.

There are actually three different herbs commonly called ginseng—Asian ginseng (*Panax ginseng*), American ginseng (*Panax quinquefolius*), and Siberian ginseng (*Eleutherococcus senticosus*). Asian ginseng, which is the focus of this chapter, is a perennial that grows in China, Korea, Japan, and the eastern part of Russia. Unfortunately, this type of ginseng is virtually extinct in its wild state; however, the herb is cultivated in many areas of Asia. American ginseng grows wild and is cultivated in the northern United States, particularly Wisconsin, and in Canada. It is the closest cousin to Asian ginseng. Siberian ginseng is a spiny bush that grows mostly in China and Siberia. It is not actually ginseng at all, but has mistakenly been labeled as such because it has similar effects to ginseng.

ACTIVE CONSTITUENTS

The primary active constituents in ginseng are called *ginsenosides*. These compounds are believed to work by stimulating the im-

The History of Ginseng

Ginseng is one of the most honored and ancient of all medicinal herbs. The Chinese extolled the virtues of the root, believing it to be a cure for many of mankind's ailments due to its "human" shape. Around 2,000 years ago, the Emperor Shen Nung, believed to be the first Chinese herbalist, described the herb as a tonic good for "harmonizing energies, removing toxic substances, brightening the eyes, and improving thought." In imperial China, fabulous prices were paid for wild ginseng root.

Petrus Jartoux, a Jesuit missionary, introduced ginseng to the Western world in the early 1700s. In the United States, serious research into the herb's possible health benefits has been conducted only since the 1940s. Much of this inquiry has evaluated a possible role for ginseng in stimulating the immune system and minimizing the effects of stress. There have even been investigations into ginseng's effects on sexual performance, although no such relationship has been found.

mune system, influencing the secretion of adrenal steroid hormones, normalizing blood sugar changes that occur in response to stress, promoting efficient metabolism, and providing some antioxidant protection for cells. So far, at least thirteen types of ginsenosides have been identified in *Panax ginseng*.

Ginseng contains other important constituents, as well, including various vitamins, minerals, and polysaccharides, long strings of sugar molecules that appear to boost immune system function.

HEALTH BENEFITS

In recent decades, ginseng has been tested in hundreds of clinical trials, many of which concluded that the herb can enhance physical performance, increase vitality, improve mental functioning, and protect against the effects of stress and aging. However, some of these studies were not scientifically designed, so the results and conclusions are not universally accepted.

Ginseng is classified pharmacologically as an adaptogenic herb, which means that it meets the following criteria: It raises the body's resistance to toxins of a physical, chemical, or biological nature; it exhibits a normalizing or balancing action in times of stress; it is harmless (or adverse reactions are very rare); and it does not influence normal body functions.

Several well-designed studies have shown that ginseng can enhance resistance to disease and boost energy levels. There was enough credible evidence for Germany's Commission E to sanction the use of ginseng for "invigoration" during times of fatigue and weakness, and for improving concentration and enhancing stamina.

In a study reported in 1996, investigators evaluated the effect of ginseng on the ability to manage everyday stress. All of the participants took a multivitamin supplement each day; half of the group also took 40 milligrams of ginseng daily. After twelve weeks, individuals in the ginseng group reported significant increases in their quality of life, while only slight improvements were reported among participants in the control group.

Another study examined ginseng's effects on the mental acuity of college-age individuals. The participants took either 200 milligrams of ginseng a day or a placebo, with no active ingredients. The group taking ginseng showed a statistically significant improvement in the speed with which they performed mathematical calculations, compared with the control group. There were no notable improvements in other cognitive abilities, however.

RECOMMENDED DOSAGE

Ginseng is available in a variety of forms, including teas, tablets, capsules, and tinctures. Most standardized extracts of Asian ginseng supply approximately 5- to 7-percent ginsenosides; the recommended dose of these extracts is 100 milligrams taken once or twice a day. Germany's Commission E recommends 1 to 2 grams of *Panax ginseng* root daily.

When you shop for ginseng products, you'll want to choose a formulation of ginseng that is made from the genus *Panax*; other forms of the herb, such as American ginseng, do not contain the same mixture of chemicals that produce the positive results associated with Asian ginseng. And, believe it or not, some "ginseng" products don't actually contain any ginseng at all—so remember to read labels carefully! Also, make sure you select a *Panax ginseng* product that's standardized to contain 5- to 7-percent ginsenosides.

Experts generally recommend the use of ginseng for up to three months at a time. However, some herbalists suggest taking ginseng for two to three weeks, followed by a two-week break during which the herb is not used.

CONSIDERATIONS FOR USE

There are no formally recognized contraindications for the use of *Panax ginseng*. However, some health-care professionals trained in herbal medicine caution that people with uncontrolled high blood pressure (hypertension) should not take the herb. Additionally, women who are pregnant or breast-feeding should not use ginseng.

Adverse side effects are very rare when ginseng is used at recommended dosage levels. There have been rare reports of nervousness, sleeplessness, diarrhea (particularly in the morning), skin rashes, and postmenopausal bleeding when the herb is taken in high doses or for long periods of time. The U.S. Food and Drug Administration has placed ginseng on its list of substances that are "Generally Recognized as Safe." However, this does not guarantee that ginseng won't cause side effects.

In 1979, *JAMA (The Journal of the American Medical Association)* published an article about "ginseng abuse syndrome" that described the side effects of long-term ginseng use as high blood pressure, anxiety and nervousness, insomnia, and skin eruptions. Most herbalists believe that the report itself was flawed, since many of the 133 people who experienced symptoms had been taking extremely high doses—up to 15 grams a day—of ginseng. Also, the commercial preparations *JAMA* reported on contained varying amounts of ginseng and were not subject to controlled analysis.

Chapter 33

Green Tea

Green tea is an ancient beverage that remains popular to this day. Worldwide, only water is consumed in greater quantities. Based on the conclusive results of some scientific studies, researchers believe that green tea can produce a number of important health benefits. Studies suggest that green tea extract may provide protection against cancer and cardiovascular disease. Although much more research needs to be done in these areas, the scientific evidence is promising.

Camellia sinensis is the scientific name for the common tea plant, a native of the rain forests of Southeast Asia. The leaf buds and young leaves of the plant are harvested to make three basic types of tea: green, oolong, and black. These are "sipping teas," which are taken primarily for the flavorful enjoyment they offer, rather than for medicinal purposes. The differences among these teas lies in the way the leaves are processed after they are picked. Green tea is unfermented; oolong is partially fermented; and black tea is fully fermented. Because some important constituents of tea may be lost during the fermenting process, unfermented tea is clearly a better source of natural chemicals. For example, green tea contains proteins, natural sugars, and vitamins that oolong and black teas do not. Many experts now believe that the substances preserved in green tea—especially the natural antioxidants—protect the body from damage by harmful free radicals. This may explain why drinking green tea can potentially protect against degenerative diseases, including cancer.

The History of Green Tea

Tea is said to have been "discovered" by the Chinese Emperor Shen Nung in 2737 BC. Legend has it that some young leaves from a wild tea bush blew unnoticed into a pot of water that the Emperor was boiling. He covered the pot and put it aside, and when he returned later to pour the water, he noticed its pleasing aroma and pale color, and took a sip . . . and a new drink was born. The accidental discovery of the beverage was later detailed by a scholar named Lu Yu in his work, *The Classic of Tea,* a Chinese scroll that dates back to AD 350.

Around AD 800, Buddhist monks introduced tea to Japan, where tea drinking evolved into a very elaborate ceremony called *cha-no-yu.* The traditional Japanese tea ceremony is of great social and religious significance. It is a time for friends to gather and socialize, and to discuss the aesthetic merits of Japanese art and calligraphy. In the proper, serene setting, this way of taking tea is said to be quite a tranquil and spiritual experience.

From Asia, the use of tea spread gradually to the rest of the world, thanks to the sixteenth century explorers and traders of the Netherlands, France, Portugal, and Britain who introduced tea to their home countries, creating a demand for the drink. Today, the tea plant is cultivated in many parts of the world, including Burma, China, India, Japan, Sri Lanka, and Africa. Green tea is the most popular beverage in Asia.

ACTIVE CONSTITUENTS

The greatest health benefits of green tea are due to the presence of plant chemicals called *polyphenols,* which are very potent antioxidants. Polyphenols protect against cardiovascular disease because they prevent the oxidation of "bad" low-density lipoprotein (LDL) cholesterol. High blood levels of LDL cholesterol have been conclusively proven to increase the risk of atherosclerosis and coronary artery disease. By preventing the oxidation of cholesterol, the polyphenols in green tea help reduce plaque buildup on the inner walls of arteries and decrease the risk of arterial blockage.

Of the polyphenols in green tea, *epigallocatechin gallate* (EGCG) ranks as the most powerful antioxidant. In animal studies, topical applications of EGCG interfered with tumor growth, suggesting that this particular phytochemical may be responsible for green tea's possible anticancer action. Some preliminary studies suggest that green tea consumption may reduce the incidence of cancers of the liver, pancreas, breast, esophagus, and lungs. More research is needed before this anticancer effect can be considered conclusively proven, but studies currently under way are producing promising results.

HEALTH BENEFITS

A study conducted at the Saitama Cancer Center Research Institute in Japan and published in the *British Medical Journal* evaluated the impact of lifestyle behaviors—including the consumption of green tea—on the health of 1,371 men over the age of forty. High tea intake was linked with a decrease in total cholesterol and triglycerides, and an increase in "good" high-density lipoprotein (HDL) cholesterol. Green tea also showed a protective effect against liver disorders. This relationship was particularly strong when green tea intake was at its highest (over ten cups per day).

Investigators at the Shanghai Cancer Institute in the People's Republic of China evaluated 734 men and women with esophageal cancer, and compared their lifestyles and dietary patterns with those of more than 1,552 people who did not have cancer. In individuals who did not drink alcohol or smoke cigarettes, green tea reduced the likelihood of developing esophageal cancer by 57 and 60 percent, respectively; the risk reductions associated with the tea were not quite as great in participants who did drink alcohol and/or use cigarettes. Overall, the more green tea consumed, the more the risk was reduced. In 1994, the researchers published the results of their study in the *Journal of the National Cancer Institute,* concluding: "Although these findings are consistent with studies in laboratory animals, indicating that green tea can inhibit esophageal carcinogenesis, further investigations are definitely needed."

RECOMMENDED DOSAGE

An optimal dose of green tea has not yet been established. As little as one or two cups of the tea taken daily appears to have a beneficial effect. However, as observed in the Saitama Center Research study, the disease-preventive ability of green tea appears to increase with an increased intake of the tea. Intakes as high as ten or more cups a day have been associated with the greatest health benefits.

Remember that polyphenols are the active ingredients responsible for many of green tea's reported health benefits. A cup of this tea can contain as much as 140 milligrams of polyphenols; however, the polyphenol levels in green tea can vary as a result of many factors, including where the tea plant was grown, how it was processed, its age, how you brewed it, and so forth.

Supplemental forms of green tea provide controlled doses of polyphenols. A capsule standardized to provide 97-percent polyphenols is equal to about four cups of green tea. Always take your green tea supplements with food and water.

CONSIDERATIONS FOR USE

Green tea has been enjoyed in many countries for thousands of years with no ill effects. Any side effects that do occur are minor, and may include stomach irritation, diarrhea, restlessness, and possibly tremors at high levels of consumption.

Chapter 34

Hawthorn

Hawthorn, known scientifically as *Crataegus oxyacantha*, is native to Europe, with closely related species found in parts of Africa and Asia. Each spring, this tree is covered with small white blossoms that yield to bright red berries during the summer. Precisely which part of the plant offers medicinal benefits is still subject to debate. Fresh and dried berries, dried flowers, and dried leaves are all used—usually in combination—in commercial preparations.

Although it is still not well known in the United States, hawthorn is enjoying increasing popularity here because of research that shows it may be helpful in the early stages of congestive heart failure. There is also some evidence that it may also improve the condition of people who have a type of chest pain known as stable angina pectoris.

ACTIVE CONSTITUENTS

Hawthorn is a rich source of *phytochemicals*—substances found in plants that may have health-promoting properties. The combined action of a number of these plant chemicals may be responsible for hawthorn's beneficial effects. *Oligomeric procyanidins* (OPCs) are a class of antioxidant phytochemicals contained in hawthorn that have a direct effect on the cardiovascular system.

Other antioxidant phytochemicals present in hawthorn are *flavonoids*. Quercetin is a flavonoid that is believed to be at least partially responsible for hawthorn's vasodilating effect.

HEALTH BENEFITS

Hawthorn appears to improve blood flow in the cardiovascular system. It may also be able to increase the strength of heart muscle contractions and lower blood pressure by dilating and reducing resistance in the blood vessels. But the strongest evidence in support of hawthorn is associated with its use in people with early-stage congestive heart failure, a condition in which the heart's pumping activity becomes inefficient, often due to a weakened heart muscle.

In 1993, German researchers reported on their study of hawthorn's effects in thirty patients, fifty to seventy years old, with early-stage congestive heart failure. The participants took either 160 milligrams of hawthorn extract or a placebo every day for eight weeks. During the course of the study, the participants also exercised regularly on a stationary bicycle. When the eight weeks were up, the individuals supplementing with hawthorn extract were able to exercise aerobically on the bicycle for a significantly longer period of time than the individuals taking the placebo. Participants in both groups showed mild declines in systolic and diastolic blood pressure.

Another study of hawthorn, published in 1983, looked at the effects of the herb on angina in sixty participants. Over the span of three weeks, the individuals involved in the study took either 180 milligrams daily of hawthorn extract or a placebo. The researchers discovered that the participants in the hawthorn group were able to exercise longer than participants in the placebo group. Tests showed increased coronary blood flow in the individuals taking hawthorn extract.

Note: Hawthorn is not meant to be a substitute for medical care in the treatment of congestive heart failure, angina, or other cardiovascular ailments. Do not use the herb without the supervision of your health-care practitioner if you have any of these heart problems.

RECOMMENDED DOSAGE

Hawthorn is available as a dried herb in capsules, fluid extract, solid extract, or tinctures. It is typically recommended in doses ranging from 160 to 900 milligrams daily, divided into two or three doses. Products are usually standardized to 18.75-percent oligo-meric procyanidins or 2.2-percent total bioflavonoids. To make hawthorn tea, simmer 1 scant teaspoon (about 1 gram) in two-thirds to 1 cup of water for fifteen minutes. Strain the tea, and it's ready to drink.

Be aware that hawthorn's actions are not immediate; some-times it may take up to six weeks before results become apparent.

CONSIDERATIONS FOR USE

Hawthorn is a very safe herb, even when used long-term. No side effects have been reported with recommended doses of the herb.

Remember that hawthorn is not meant as a substitute for med-ical intervention in the case of heart ailments.

Chapter 35

Horse Chestnut

The horse chestnut tree, *Aesculus hippocastanum*, is indigenous to northern and central Asia, but today is widely cultivated in many European countries, and is commonly found in England. It has been suggested that the plant gets its curious name from the unusual imprints resembling tiny horseshoes that cover its branches. In truth, these are leaf scars, which mark the spots where leaves once grew from the tree's branches.

Traditionally, the horse chestnut tree was grown largely for ornamental purposes, and today it is still planted in parks or in private gardens, where it can be admired during the spring, burgeoning with white blossoms. Researchers have found that the fruit of the tree—the chestnut itself—may contain medicinal properties. Most notably, an extract from the horse chestnut may promote the health of circulatory vessels. In recent years, this extract has become a popular alternative treatment for disorders of the leg veins.

ACTIVE CONSTITUENTS

A number of active chemicals in horse chestnut have so far been identified. The primary constituent is a complex mixture known as *aescin*, which has anti-inflammatory characteristics. Aescin has also been shown to reduce edema, the accumulation of fluid in body tissues, and appears to be particularly useful in enhancing the tone of the veins, as well. It not only acts as a diuretic, but also reduces enzyme activity that contributes to fluid buildup.

HEALTH BENEFITS

In Germany, horse chestnut has been formally approved for the treatment of chronic venous insufficiency and related symptoms, such as pain or heaviness in the legs, cramps in the calves, and swelling and itching of the legs. The herb is also used in the treatment of both superficial and deep varicose veins.

German researchers at the University of Heidelberg examined the effects of horse chestnut on edema of the legs due to venous insufficiency in 240 participants. One group of participants took a horse chestnut supplement containing 50 milligrams of aescin twice daily; individuals in a second group were asked to wear compression stockings every day; and a third group of participants took a placebo daily. The results of the study, published in *The Lancet* in 1996, showed that horse chestnut does, indeed, promote the health of the leg veins. After twelve weeks of therapy, measurements of lower leg volume showed, on average, a 25 percent reduction of edema in participants taking horse chestnut, as well as in the individuals wearing compression stockings. No changes were observed in the placebo group.

Data from thirteen studies of horse chestnut were combined and evaluated by researchers at the University of Exeter in the United Kingdom. The researchers found that horse chestnut was consistently superior to placebos in patients with chronic venous insufficiency. Horse chestnut produced decreases in lower-leg volume and in leg circumference (at the calf and ankle). It also eased leg pain, itching, and feelings of tension and fatigue, symptoms that are commonly associated with venous insufficiency. In an article published in *Archives of Dermatology* in 1998, the investigators concluded that horse chestnut "represents a treatment option for [chronic venous insufficiency] that is worth considering."

RECOMMENDED DOSAGE

A typical recommended dose of horse chestnut extract is the equivalent of 90 to 150 milligrams of aescin per day. Once improvement is seen, the dosage can be reduced to the equivalent of 35 to 70 milligrams.

CONSIDERATIONS FOR USE

Occasional side effects may occur with horse chestnut, including itching, nausea, and upset stomach. These are very rare when horse chestnut is taken at the recommended dosage level.

Chapter 36

Kava

The kava plant is a member of the pepper family that's indigenous to the islands of the South Pacific, including Hawaii, Papua New Guinea, Fiji, Samoa, and Tahiti. This eight- to ten-foot-tall shrub is covered with large, heart-shaped leaves. Its tough roots contain the active ingredients.

The South Pacific islanders sometimes refer to kava (also called kava-kava) as the "root of tranquility." For the past three thousand years, the herb has been used by the islands' residents for its soothing, calming effects. Scientifically, kava is known as *Piper methysticum,* which literally means "intoxicating pepper." In many parts of the world, the herb is now used to relieve anxiety.

ACTIVE CONSTITUENTS

Kava's calming effects seem to be due to the action of fat-like compounds called *kavalactones,* which are contained in the root of the plant. They appear to have a soothing influence on the nervous system, producing muscle relaxation and sleep. In fact, their activity has been compared with that of benzodiazepines, prescription medications that are used to relieve anxiety. The highest quality roots are believed to have a kavalactone content of up to eight percent.

HEALTH BENEFITS

Germany's Commission E has approved kava for the treatment of

The History of Kava

Kava has been an important part of the many cultures of the South Pacific Islands for centuries. Traditionally, beverages made from the kava root, often mixed with coconut milk or water, have been consumed before the evening meal. To this day, it is customary for the islanders to drink kava as part of religious, community, and social occasions. Many different occasions—from informal gatherings to religious rites—are still marked by the ceremonial drinking of kava served in a halved coconut shell.

During the late nineteenth century and the early part of the twentieth century, German herbalists prescribed kava-based syrups for a variety of ailments, including high blood pressure. By 1914, it was added to the *British Pharmacopoeia* under the name "kava rhizoma," and as its therapeutic properties became known, its use spread to the United States, where it is prescribed as a mild sedative.

anxiety, restlessness, and stress. Nevertheless, the amount of carefully conducted research on kava is still limited, and almost all of the studies have been conducted by European investigators.

The largest study of kava, published in the journal *Pharmacopsychiatry* in 1997, was conducted at Jena University in Germany. Researchers studied kava's effects on 101 people with anxiety-related disorders. Over the course of twenty-five weeks, the participants took either 100 milligrams of a 70-percent kavalactone extract three times daily or a placebo with no active ingredients. Anxiety levels decreased in both the kava and the placebo groups; however, the decreases were more significant in the participants taking the herb. There were no differences in side effects between the groups, and those taking the herb did not experience any of the negative effects often associated with benzodiazepines, such as decreased mental capacity and slower reaction time.

Kava has been claimed to have other benefits, such as the ability to ease menopausal symptoms, but research in these areas has been scarce and inconclusive.

RECOMMENDED DOSAGE

The recommended dose of kava is equivalent to 60 to 120 milligrams of kavalactones per day. Positive effects may not become apparent until after two weeks of use.

CONSIDERATIONS FOR USE

Women who are pregnant or breast-feeding should not take kava. Also, the herb should not be taken at the same time as any drugs that act on the central nervous system, including benzodiazepines, antidepressants, barbiturates, and alcohol.

High doses of kava taken over long periods of time can cause impaired motor reflexes and a temporary yellowing of the skin, nails, and hair. Very rarely, allergic skin reactions may occur.

Chapter 37

Milk Thistle

Milk thistle, or *Silybum marianum,* is a prickly herb covered with spines that thrives in dry, rocky soils of southern and western Europe and in some parts of the United States. The plant has a branched stem that can reach a height of up to three feet, and each stalk is topped with a purple flower. Its leaves are a dark, glossy green with spiny edges and milk-white veins. For over 2,000 years, the seeds, fruit, and leaves of the milk thistle have been used for their medicinal benefits.

Traditionally, milk thistle has been used to treat disorders of the liver. In the early 1600s, herbalist Nicholas Culpepper recommended the herb to remove "obstructions" of the liver, and suggested using the fresh root and seeds to treat jaundice. Today, milk thistle is sometimes called the "liver herb," because it contains active constituents that protect liver cells from chemical damage, and may improve the function of liver cells that have already been injured. According to scientific evidence, milk thistle may be very valuable in the treatment of jaundice, hepatitis, and alcoholic cirrhosis.

ACTIVE CONSTITUENTS

A complex of chemicals, collectively called *silymarin,* are the active constituents that give milk thistle its medicinal properties. These chemicals, of which *silibilin* is the most potent, protect and stabilize the membranes of liver cells by attaching to receptor sites on the membranes; this prevents toxic substances, such as alcohol, from penetrating liver cells.

There is also evidence that silymarin is a powerful antioxidant that protects liver cells against free-radical damage. Everyday, we are exposed to toxic chemicals—cigarette smoke, car exhaust, and pesticides, among others—that cause the production of free radicals, the reactive molecules that wreak havoc on healthy cells and tissues, including those of the liver. Silymarin greatly enhances the activity of two of the body's natural antioxidants, glutathione peroxidase and superoxide dismutase (SOD), and heightens the body's defense against the effects of toxic chemicals.

In addition, the active constituents in milk thistle increase protein synthesis in liver cells, including the synthesis of DNA and RNA, the body's genetic material. Because of this action, milk thistle promotes the production of new liver cells to replace old or damaged cells, and may reverse symptoms of both acute and chronic liver problems.

HEALTH BENEFITS

Milk thistle is widely used in the treatment of both chronic and acute liver disorders; it is especially beneficial as a therapy for alcohol-related liver disease. Although milk thistle is typically not considered a frontline treatment for viral hepatitis, it can be used to complement the medical management of the illness, especially when the condition is chronic and active. Studies of the herb's effects on liver damage due to alcohol, viruses, or exposure to toxins have proven that the herb has significant protective and restorative actions.

Researchers at the University of Vienna examined milk thistle's effects on advanced cirrhosis of the liver in 170 participants. About half of the participants took silymarin, while the other half took a placebo, with no active ingredients. The patients' progress was tracked over the course of three to six years. The researchers found that individuals taking silymarin showed improvements in liver function. More significant, however, was the fact that 58 percent of the milk-thistle group survived the entire duration of the study, compared with only 39 percent of the placebo group. Milk thistle was more effective in the treatment of alcohol-related cirrhosis than in the treatment of cirrhosis caused by other factors.

In contrast, a study conducted at the University of Spain in Barcelona failed to find any positive evidence of milk thistle's medicinal benefits for people with alcoholic cirrhosis. For this study, 200 patients took either milk thistle or a placebo over a two-year period. The results showed that the course of the disease was not significantly affected in either group, and that individuals in the milk-thistle group did not have a higher survival rate than those in the placebo group.

Interestingly, a number of studies have evaluated the use of milk thistle in people who consumed *Amanita phalloides*, known as Avenging Angel mushrooms, which contain highly toxic alkaloids. Milk thistle extract was found to prevent liver damage when it was given intravenously within the first day after the mushrooms were eaten, particularly if administered within the first few hours. In one study of sixty patients who were treated with milk thistle for *Amanita* poisoning, all survived; other studies of untreated individuals have shown a 50 percent mortality rate in these people.

Note: Liver disease is a very serious condition—it is not an illness that should be self-treated. Medical supervision is essential in the treatment of any liver disorder.

RECOMMENDED DOSAGE

The recommended dosage of milk thistle extract is 140 milligrams three times a day of an extract standardized to 70- to 80-percent silymarin complex. If improvement is noted after several weeks of therapy, the dosage can be decreased to 280 milligrams daily.

CONSIDERATIONS FOR USE

Very few side effects have been reported with the use of milk thistle, and have generally been limited to gastrointestinal discomfort, including loose stools or diarrhea, during the initial two to three days of treatment. Side effects usually subside after these first few days, as the body becomes more accustomed to the herb.

Chapter 38

St. John's Wort

St. John's wort, or *Hypericum perforatum,* is a perennial that grows up to three feet tall, with pale green leaves and bright yellow flowers. The plant is native to many parts of Europe and Asia. Its common name comes from the early Christians, who renamed *Hypericum perforatum* after St. John the Baptist, because it was traditionally collected on St. John's Day. "Wort" is simply the Old English word for "plant." The medicinal properties of this herb are contained in its leaves and flowers.

In recent years, St. John's wort has been called "nature's Prozac" because research has shown it to be an effective treatment for mild to moderate depression in many people—without the side effects often associated with prescription antidepressants. The herb is the treatment of choice in many European countries, and since an estimated 17 million American adults are affected by depression every year, it's no wonder St. John's wort has been attracting so much attention in the United States, as well.

ACTIVE CONSTITUENTS

The medicinal benefits of St. John's wort have been attributed to a combination of active ingredients, including flavonoids, bioflavones, hypericins, and xanthones. Nevertheless, the precise mechanism by which the herb functions as an antidepressant has not yet been defined. Some early studies suggested that the herb interferes with the production of an enzyme called *monoamine oxidase* (MAO), which affects brain chemicals associated with mood and

The History of St. John's Wort

The earliest records of the use of St. John's wort date back to Greek and Roman times. It was a known treatment for a wide variety of ailments, ranging from lung disorders to depression, and was also used to heal injuries, such as wounds, burns, and bruises. The herb was also believed to have mystical powers. In fact, it was named *Hypericum* from the Greek meaning "to overcome an apparition," referring to its reputed ability to protect against evil spirits. During the Middle Ages, people often placed St. John's wort under their pillows at night, believing that it would fend off evil spirits and even death itself.

When the colonists came to the New World, they brought St. John's wort with them. But the herb fell out of favor in the United States during the latter part of the nineteenth century and into the twentieth century—as did many herbal remedies—due largely to the emergence of pharmaceutical products. More recently, St. John's wort has been rediscovered, and has enjoyed a revival in the last several decades. In Europe, it is often taken as a tea to calm anxiety and ease depression. Reports from Germany indicate that physicians there recommend the herb more often than they prescribe Prozac. As studies have shown St. John's wort to be effective in the treatment of mild to moderate depression, sales of the herb in the United States have increased twentyfold from 1995 to 1997.

depression; however, this has not been proven in humans. More recently, attention has turned to a neurotransmitter in the brain called *serotonin*, which is believed to promote well-being and is present in low amounts in depressed individuals. Like prescription antidepressants, such as fluoxetine (Prozac), sertraline (Zoloft), and paroxetine (Paxil), St. John's wort appears to increase levels of serotonin in the brain.

HEALTH BENEFITS

Scientific research has led to the widespread use of St. John's wort as an antidepressant in some European countries. A study published in the *Journal of Geriatric Psychiatry and Neurology* in 1994 reported on the effects of the herb on depression in 135 individuals. One group of participants took 300 milligrams three times daily of St. John's wort extract, while a second group took 25 milligrams three times daily of the prescription tricyclic antidepressant drug imipramine (Tofranil). After four weeks, both groups showed comparable improvements in depression levels, with declines noted on three separate scales used to measure depression; however, the participants taking St. John's wort experienced fewer and milder side effects.

In a review published in the *British Medical Journal* in 1996, researchers in the United States and Germany examined the results of twenty-three existing European studies of St. John's wort, involving a total of more than 1,700 people with depression. Fifteen of the twenty-three studies compared the effects of St. John's wort extract with those of a placebo, and concluded that symptoms improved in 55 percent of the individuals taking the herb, compared with 22 percent of the individuals taking a placebo. The remaining eight studies compared the effects of St. John's wort with low-dose prescription antidepressants, such as amitriptyline (Elavil) and imipramine (Tofranil). In these studies, a slightly greater number of the participants taking the herb improved—64 percent of individuals taking St. John's wort, compared with 59 percent of those taking prescription medications. The researchers also reported that 20 percent of the participants taking St. John's wort experienced side effects, compared with 36 percent of the individuals taking prescription antidepressants.

Although these studies are encouraging, some researchers have noted that most trials of St. John's wort have involved relatively few patients and have lasted only a few weeks. The National Institutes of Health recently began the first large-scale clinical trial of St. John's wort, involving patients with major depression. The results of this trial should help clarify the herb's efficacy in treating depression.

Note: If you are severely depressed and unable to function in day-to-day tasks, or if you have thoughts of suicide, consult a physician for immediate treatment.

RECOMMENDED DOSAGE

St. John's wort is most commonly taken in tablet and capsule form. The recommended dosage of the herb extract is 300 milligrams, taken three times daily. When you choose a product, look for an extract that is standardized to contain 0.3-percent hypericin. Many people also take St. John's wort as a tea, although you should be aware that there has been much less research conducted on the effects of the herb taken in tea form. To prepare the tea, steep 1 to 2 teaspoonfuls of the dried, finely chopped herb in about two-thirds of a cup of hot water for ten minutes. Drink 1 to 2 cups of the tea daily.

At the present time, most herbalists recommend the use of St. John's wort for mild to moderate depression only. Experts caution that it may take four to six weeks after starting therapy with the herb before results become apparent.

CONSIDERATIONS FOR USE

Women who are pregnant or breast-feeding should not take St. John's wort, because research on its safety in the unborn and in infants is still very limited. Also, people who take prescription antidepressants should not stop using these medications, change their dosage, or switch to St. John's wort without their doctor's consent and supervision.

Because of possible interactions, St. John's wort should not be taken in combination with amphetamines. Also, be cautious about drinking alcohol when using the herb.

Side effects associated with the use of St. John's wort include indigestion, allergic reactions, fatigue, and restlessness. The herb may cause phototoxicity, or increased sensitivity to light, in some individuals taking high doses—particularly in those who are fair-skinned. To date, most studies have been conducted over the short-term (no longer than six weeks), and thus information on side effects during long-term use is not available.

Chapter 39

Saw Palmetto

S aw palmetto, or *Serenoa repens*, is a small palm tree that grows up to 8 to 10 feet high, and is indigenous to the southeastern coastal states of North America. The tree has large, fan-like leaves and reddish- to brownish-black berries. Extracts from saw palmetto berries have been studied for their benefits in treating disorders of the prostate gland.

The prostate is located at the base of the bladder, surrounding both the urethra and the ejaculatory duct. It produces fluids that combine with sperm from the testicles and other secretions to form semen, and acts as a valve that permits both semen and urine to flow in the proper direction. *Benign prostatic hyperplasia* (BPH) is the nonmalignant enlargement of the prostate gland that primarily affects men over fifty. The incidence of this disorder increases with age. Prostate enlargement compresses the urethra and restricts the flow of urine out of the bladder, resulting in a reduction in the size and force of the urine stream, difficulty starting urine flow, and frequent nighttime urination.

As positive evidence accumulates about the benefits of saw palmetto for prostate health, its use in BPH and other prostate disorders is becoming more widespread.

ACTIVE CONSTITUENTS

Although the exact cause of BPH is still not clearly understood, researchers believe that prostatic enlargement is hormone induced.

The History of Saw Palmetto

As far back as the early 1700s, Native Americans in the southeastern United States used saw palmetto berries to treat swelling and inflammation of the prostate gland. They also made use of the herb as a therapy for erectile dysfunction. The herb was included in the *National Formulary,* a pharmacist's reference guide, until 1950; mention of saw palmetto was removed when the herb's efficacy was called into question by some scientists.

Saw palmetto is accepted in Germany as a treatment for benign prostate enlargement, and it is sold over-the-counter for that purpose. With the renewed interest in natural treatments for medical disorders, saw palmetto is becoming more well known in America.

Specifically, the abnormal growth of the prostate may occur because of the presence of *dihydrotestosterone* (DHT), a metabolite of the sex hormone testosterone.

Researchers believe that phytosterols and free fatty acids, which are present in saw palmetto berries, block the formation of DHT, and thus inhibit prostatic enlargement. Extracts of saw palmetto may also inhibit certain substances that lead to inflammation, irritation, and smooth muscle spasms in the prostate gland. Irritation and spasm of the smooth muscles of the prostate and urethra initiate the urgency and frequency of urination experienced with BPH.

HEALTH BENEFITS

Most of the existing studies of saw palmetto have been conducted in Europe. Although research in the United States has been limited, the results of some studies have been promising. One six-month-long study of moderate BPH in 1,098 men over age fifty compared the effects of saw palmetto with finasteride (Proscar), a prescription medication for BPH. In 1996, the researchers reported their results in the journal *Prostate*, concluding that both treatments relieved BPH symptoms in about two-thirds of the patients. There were significant improvements in peak urinary flow rate in both groups—an increase average of 25 percent in the saw palmetto group, compared with 30 percent in the finasteride group.

Researchers at the Minneapolis Veterans Affairs Medical Center and other institutions conducted a review and analysis of eighteen previously conducted studies of saw palmetto extract, involving a total of 2,939 men. Their results—published in *JAMA (The Journal of the American Medical Association)* in 1998—showed that treatment with saw palmetto extract reduced BPH symptoms by about 28 percent and improved peak urinary flow rate by about 24 percent. Furthermore, the men taking saw palmetto were twice as likely to experience improvements in their symptoms as men in the placebo groups.

RECOMMENDED DOSAGE

Saw palmetto is available in a variety of forms, including whole berries, powders made from whole berries, liquid extracts such as tinctures, concentrates, extracts, and standardized extracts. The recommended daily dosage is 1 to 2 grams of saw palmetto berries, or 320 milligrams of the lipophilic (fat-soluble) extract. Be aware that six to eight weeks of treatment may be necessary before benefits become apparent.

CONSIDERATIONS FOR USE

Because saw palmetto is believed to act on sex hormones, including estrogen, pregnant women and women of childbearing age should not use the herb.

Saw palmetto has no known negative interactions with drugs or dietary supplements. Side effects may include mild stomach upset and/or headaches; these reactions occur very rarely, however.

Chapter 40

Valerian

Valerian, also known as the garden heliotrope, is a perennial plant that grows up to four feet tall, bearing feathery leaves and pink flowers. *Valeriana officinales,* as valerian is called scientifically, thrives in damp meadowlands and along riverbanks. The plant is known to have a distinctive, unpleasant aroma.

The root of the valerian plant is considered to be medicinally valuable, and it has traditionally been used for its tranquilizing properties and sedative action. Today, valerian is commonly used by people who suffer from insomnia as an alternative to prescription sleeping aids.

ACTIVE CONSTITUENTS

Studies have shown that valerian has a depressive effect on the central nervous system, but the specific site of action and the particular constituents responsible for this effect have not yet been defined. At one time, scientists believed that compounds called *valepotriates* were responsible for valerian's therapeutic effects; however, more recent studies have raised doubts about the role of these substances.

Valerian contains many other phytochemicals, including sesquiterpenes, alkaloids, and caffeic-acid derivatives, but researchers have been unable to identify which ingredient, or specific combination of ingredients, is responsible for the therapeutic effects of valerian.

The History of Valerian

In medieval times, many herbalists called valerian "all-cure," believing that the herb could be used to cure virtually any ailment. It was commonly recommended as a decongestant, a diuretic, and a pain-reliever. By the seventeenth century, there were also claims that the herb could protect against the plague, and it was used as a treatment for coughs and menstrual discomfort.

During World War I, valerian was taken by many Europeans suffering from "bombing neurosis," who were anxious and shell-shocked from their exposure to artillery bombardment. The herb was listed until 1950 in the *National Formulary,* a guide for pharmacists. Valerian has been called the "Valium of the nineteenth century," and is becoming popular again as a natural remedy for anxiety, nervousness, and insomnia. It is a common ingredient in over-the-counter sleeping aids sold in Europe.

HEALTH BENEFITS

Several studies have shown that valerian has sedative properties, and is capable of inducing and maintaining sleep, as well as improving its quality. These benefits were confirmed in a double-blind Swedish study published in 1989, in which a 400-milligram dose of valerian was compared with a placebo. Of the thirty subjects who participated in the study, twenty-four rated the valerian preparation better than the placebo, two considered the effects to be equal, and four thought the placebo produced better results. No side effects were observed from use of the herb.

In a separate study of 128 people, researchers asked participants to alternate between taking 400 milligrams of valerian root extract and a placebo. When using valerian, the volunteers fell asleep more rapidly, and the quality of their sleep was much better than while they were taking the placebo. The improvement in sleep quality due to the use of valerian was particularly strong in those individuals who had considered themselves poor sleepers and who were smokers. Valerian did not cause side effects such as nighttime awakenings, nor did it have a negative impact on dream recall.

Despite these positive findings, most experts agree that more carefully structured studies are needed to clearly define valerian's effects.

RECOMMENDED DOSAGE

Valerian is available in a number of forms, including extracts, tinctures, and teas. For extracts, the recommended dosage is equivalent to 2 to 3 grams of valerian, taken one or more times daily. For tinctures, one-half to 1 teaspoon should be taken one or more times per day. If you prefer taking valerian as a tea, try 2 to 3 grams (or 1 teaspoon per cup) of the herb one or more times daily.

CONSIDERATIONS FOR USE

When valerian is used at recommended dosage levels, side effects are very rare. With higher doses or long-term use, there have been occasional reports of headaches, stomach upset, sleeplessness, and restlessness.

Conclusion

G reat care has been taken to ensure that the information in this book is up-to-date and accurate. But one thing is certain: Much of it will change in the future, because literally thousands of scientific studies of vitamins, minerals, herbs, and other supplements are underway at this time. Some studies will validate and confirm what we believe to be true about nutrients. Others, however, will disprove some existing theories. If this seems disconcerting, you can take some comfort from the fact that—in the long run—continuous and ongoing scientific reevaluation actually serves to protect you.

While the focus of this book is on vitamins, minerals, and herbs, you should be aware that many studies currently in progress are examining the possible health-promoting benefits of other nutritional supplements, such as soy protein and glucosamine. The FDA now recognizes the value of soy protein, and is allowing the claim that taking 25 grams of soy protein daily (as part of a diet that is low in saturated fat and cholesterol) will lower cholesterol levels and reduce your risk of heart disease. And the Arthritis Association has recognized the benefits that glucosamine offers to some people who have osteoarthritis.

I believe that ongoing research will ultimately lead to the acceptance of similar kinds of health claims for other nutrients, including fish oils and grape-seed extract. In the meantime, you can expect to be confronted with hundreds—if not thousands—of other marketing campaigns for nutritional supplements. Some of these claims will be supported by statistically valid scientific studies; others will not. So how do you tell the difference? As a rule, be cautious—but maintain an open mind. Don't race out to purchase a "breakthrough" product that promises miracles. And don't try any supplement unless there is *reliable scientific evidence* that it works and is safe.

Examine not only the scientific evidence, but look closely at the source of the information. Generally speaking, you can trust large studies conducted at reputable academic institutions, especially when the results have been confirmed by separate studies at other institutions or organizations. But you should question small, single studies conducted by the supplement manufacturers themselves; these studies are rarely subjected to adequate outside inspection and review. Also, it's best to avoid products that are backed by "testimonials" from individual users—this kind of anecdotal evidence has no scientific value.

Ask both your physician and your pharmacist about any new supplements you are considering using. A health professional can tell you if a supplement is appropriate for your particular needs, or if it may actually be inappropriate—for example, because of a potential adverse interaction with a drug you are taking.

Remember that a nutritional approach should *complement* the medical care and advice you get from your doctor. A balanced, wholesome diet should be the foundation of your nutritional program, and nutritional supplements should serve only to enrich an already healthful lifestyle, not to compensate for poor health habits. This is one of the most important things you can do to achieve lifelong good health.

Appendix A

Nutrient Tables

By now you know that—for your health's sake—you should be striving to maximize your intake of the essential vitamins and minerals. This can be easy, if you know which foods and beverages are good sources of the nutrients you need to achieve optimal health and life-long wellness. The tables included in this appendix are meant to guide you in selecting nutrient-rich foods to make the most of your diet. Don't forget: It's best to rely on dietary sources for the vitamins and minerals you need. Use nutritional supplements as necessary to complement a healthful diet and wholesome lifestyle.

Table A.1. Good Sources of Vitamin A

Food or Beverage	Vitamin A (micrograms of RE)	Food or Beverage	Vitamin A (micrograms of RE)
American cheese (1 ounce)	82	Hubbard squash, baked (1/2 cup)	616
Apricots, raw (3 medium)	277	Ice cream, vanilla (1 cup)	133
Asparagus, boiled (1/2 cup)	75	Kale, boiled (1/2 cup)	481
Avocado, Florida (1/2 medium)	93	Lobster, cooked (3 ounces)	74
Beef liver, braised (3 1/2 ounces)	10,602	Mackerel, raw (3 ounces)	140
Beet greens, boiled (1/2 cup)	367	Mango (1 medium)	806
Broccoli, boiled (1/2 cup)	110	Milk, 1% (1 cup)	145
Butter (1 tablespoon)	114	Muenster cheese (1 ounce)	90
Butternut squash, boiled (1/2 cup)	714	Mustard greens, boiled (1/2 cup)	212
Camembert cheese (1 ounce)	71	Nectarine (1 medium)	100
Cantaloupe (1 cup)	516	Oatmeal, instant (1 packet)	455
Carrot (1 medium)	2,025	Parsley (1/2 cup)	156
Carrot juice, canned (6 ounces)	4,738	Provolone cheese (1 ounce)	75
Cheddar cheese (1 ounce)	86	Prunes, dried (10 prunes)	167
Chicken liver, simmered (3 1/2 ounces)	4,913	Pumpkin, boiled (1/2 cup)	132
Clams (4 large or 9 small)	255	Ricotta cheese, part-skim (1/2 cup)	140
Colby cheese (1 ounce)	78	Sweet potato, baked (1 medium)	2,488
Collard greens, boiled (1 cup)	349	Swiss chard, boiled (1/2 cup)	276
Cream of Wheat, instant (1 packet)	375	Swiss cheese (1 ounce)	72
Cream cheese (1 ounce)	124	Swordfish, raw (3 ounces)	101
Egg, boiled (1 large)	78	Tangerine (1 medium)	77
Guava (1 medium)	71	Tomato (1 medium)	139
Halibut, raw (3 ounces)	132	Tomato juice, canned (6 ounces)	101
Herring, raw (3 ounces)	80	Turnip greens, boiled (1/2 cup)	213

Table A.2. Good Sources of Carotenoids

Food or Beverage	Carotenoids (milligrams)	Food or Beverage	Carotenoids (milligrams)
Apricot		Lettuce, romaine (1 cup)	1.06
canned, drained (1/2 cup)	1.70	Mango (1/2 medium)	1.33
dried (7 halves)	4.31		
fresh (4 medium)	17.62	Mustard greens (1 cup)	1.51
Broccoli, boiled (1/2 cup)	1.01	Peach, dried (1 peach)	2.31
Cantaloupe (1 cup)	4.80	Pepper, red (1 cup)	3.30
Carrot, raw (1 cup)	10.82	Pumpkin (1/2 cup)	2.70
Chicory leaf, raw (1 cup)	6.17	Spinach	
Collard greens (1 cup)	10.04	cooked, drained (1/2 cup)	4.95
Cress, leaf, raw (1 cup)	2.08	raw (1 cup)	2.30
Fennel leaves (1 cup)	4.01	Winter squash, cooked (1/2 cup)	3.69
Grapefruit, pink (1/2 medium)	1.57	Sweet potato, baked (1/3 cup)	3.99
Guava (1/2 cup)	1.00	Swiss chard (1 cup)	1.31
Kale (1 cup)	3.20	Tomato juice, canned (1 cup)	2.20
Leek, raw (1 cup)	1.04	Tomato sauce, canned (1/2 cup)	1.23

Table A.3. Good Sources of Vitamin D

Food or Beverage	Vitamin D (IU)	Food or Beverage	Vitamin D (IU)
Bran Flakes cereal (3/4 cup)	50	Margarine (1 tablespoon)	60
Cod liver oil (1 tablespoon)	1,145.6	Milk, vitamin-D fortified	
Corn Flakes cereal (1 cup)	50	(1 cup)	100.0
Egg (1 large)	36.4	Sardines, canned (3 ounces)	255.2
Herring, grilled (3 ounces)	850.4	Special K cereal (1 1/3 cup)	50
Mackerel, fried (3 ounces)	718.0	Tuna, canned in oil (3 ounces)	197.2

Table A.4. Good Sources of Vitamin E

Food or Beverage	Vitamin E (IU)	Food or Beverage	Vitamin E (IU)
Almond oil (1 tablespoon)	8.16	Ranch dressing (1 tablespoon)*	3.75
Almonds (1/4 cup)	11.33	Russian dressing (1/4 tablespoon)*	5.70
Canola oil (1 tablespoon)	13.47	Safflower oil (1 tablespoon)	7.76
Cashews (1/2 cup)	3.86	Sesame oil (1 tablespoon)	5.91
Corn oil (1 tablespoon)	21.21	Skim milk (1 cup)	11.25
Cottonseed oil (1 tablespoon)	13.26	Soybean oil (1 tablespoon)	21.21
Filberts (1/4 cup)	12.11	Soybeans, boiled (1/2 cup)	8.85
French dressing (1 tablespoon)*	6.60	Sunflower oil (1 tablespoon)	12.86
Hazelnuts (1/4 cup)	12.11	Sunflower seeds (1/4 cup)	10.95
Italian dressing (1 tablespoon)*	6.60	Sweet potato, baked (1 medium)	7.80
Kale, cooked (1/2 cup)	4.02	Thousand island dressing (1 tablespoon)*	7.50
Macadamia nuts (1/4 cup)	8.25		
Milk, whole (1 cup)	11.55	Tofu (1/2 cup)	6.30
Oil and vinegar dressing (1 tablespoon)*	4.50	Wheat germ, toasted (1/4 cup)	11.66
		Wheat germ oil (1 tablespoon)	52.02
Palm oil (1 tablespoon)	5.31	Wild rice (1 cup)	4.80
Peanut oil (1 tablespoon)	3.75		
Peanuts (1/4 cup)	5.48		

* The vitamin E content of most low-calorie dressings is substantially lower.

Table A.5. Good Sources of Vitamin K

Food or Beverage	Vitamin K (micrograms)	Food or Beverage	Vitamin K (micrograms)
Asparagus, raw (1 cup)	52.26	Green cabbage (1/2 cup)	52.15
Beef liver (3 ounces)	88.45	Green tea (1 cup)	1,686.02
Broccoli, raw (1 cup)	116.16	Lentils, dry (3 1/2 ounces)	223.00
Chicken liver (3 ounces)	68.04	Peas, dry (3 1/2 ounces)	81.00
Coffee (1 cup)	89.98	Pork liver (3 ounces)	74.84
Egg (1 extra large)	28.80	Soybeans, raw (3 1/2 ounces)	190.00
Garbanzo beans, dry (3 1/2 ounces)	264.00	Spinach, raw (1 cup)	148.96
		Turnip greens, raw (1/2 cup)	148.75

Table A.6. Good Sources of Thiamin

Food or Beverage	Thiamin (milligrams)	Food or Beverage	Thiamin (milligrams)
Baker's yeast, dry (1 ounce)	0.66	Navy beans, boiled (1 cup)	0.37
Black beans, boiled (1 cup)	0.42	Oatmeal, instant (1 packet)	0.53
Black-eyed peas, boiled (1 cup)	0.35	Pinto beans, boiled (1 cup)	0.32
Brazil nuts (1 ounce)	0.28	Pork	
Brewer's yeast (1 ounce)	4.43	loin, roasted (3$^1/_2$ ounces)	0.61
Ham, canned (3$^1/_2$ ounces)	0.96	shoulder, roasted (3$^1/_2$ ounces)	0.54
Kidney beans, boiled (1 cup)	0.28	Sunflower seeds, dried (1 ounce)	0.65
Lentils, boiled (1 cup)	0.34	Trout, raw (3 ounces)	0.30
Lima beans, boiled (1 cup)	0.30	Wheat germ, toasted ($^1/_4$ cup)	0.47

Table A.7. Good Sources of Riboflavin

Food or Beverage	Riboflavin (milligrams)	Food or Beverage	Riboflavin (milligrams)
Almonds (1 ounce)	0.22	Ice milk, vanilla (1 cup)	0.35
Anchovies, raw (3 ounces)	0.22	Lamb, leg of, roasted (3 ounces)	0.23
Baker's yeast (1 ounce)	1.53	Mackerel, raw (3 ounces)	0.27
Beef		Milk, 1% (1 cup)	0.41
bottom round, braised (3$^1/_2$ ounces)	0.25	Miso ($^1/_2$ cup)	0.35
liver, braised (3$^1/_2$ ounces)	4.10	Oatmeal, instant (1 packet)	0.29
top round, broiled (3$^1/_2$ ounces)	0.26	Peaches, dried (10 halves)	0.28
Beet greens, boiled ($^1/_2$ cup)	0.21	Pears, dried (10 halves)	0.25
Brewer's yeast (1 ounce)	1.21	Pork	
Buttermilk (1 cup)	0.38	loin, roasted (3$^1/_2$ ounces)	0.32
Chicken		shoulder, roasted (3$^1/_2$ ounces)	0.32
dark meat, roasted (3$^1/_2$ ounces)	0.21	Ricotta cheese, part-skim ($^1/_2$ cup)	0.23
liver, simmered (3$^1/_2$ ounces)	1.75	Salmon, raw (3 ounces)	0.32
Cottage cheese, low-fat (8 ounces)	0.37	Trout, raw (3 ounces)	0.28
Ham, canned (3$^1/_2$ ounces)	0.23	Turkey, dark meat, roasted (3$^1/_2$ ounces)	0.24
Herring, raw (3 ounces)	0.20	Wheat germ, toasted ($^1/_2$ cup)	0.23
Ice cream, vanilla (1 cup)	0.33	Yogurt, low-fat (8 ounces)	0.40

Table A.8. Good Sources of Niacin

Food or Beverage	Niacin (milligrams)	Food or Beverage	Niacin (milligrams)
Anchovies, raw (3 ounces)	11.9	Ham, canned (3½ ounces)	3.2
Beef		Lamb	
bottom round, braised (3½ ounces)	3.9	loin chop, broiled (1 chop)	3.1
brisket, braised (3½ ounces)	3.0	rib chop, broiled (1 chop)	3.6
flank steak, broiled (3½ ounces)	4.8	leg of, roasted (3 ounces)	4.7
ground, lean, baked (3½ ounces)	4.3	Mackerel, raw (3 ounces)	7.4
liver, braised (3½ ounces)	10.7	Oatmeal, instant (1 packet)	5.5
top round, broiled (3½ ounces)	5.9	Peaches, dried (10 halves)	5.7
Chicken		Peanuts (1 ounce)	4.0
breast meat, roasted (½ breast)	12.5	Pork	
dark and light meat, roasted (3½ ounces)	8.5	loin, roasted (3½ ounces)	5.4
dark meat only, roasted (3½ ounces)	6.4	shoulder, roasted (3½ ounces)	4.0
leg meat, roasted (1 leg)	7.1	Salmon (3 ounces, raw)	6.7
light meat, roasted (3½ ounces)	11.1	Tuna, canned in water (3 ounces)	4.9
liver, simmered (3½ ounces)	4.5	Turkey	
thigh meat, roasted (1 thigh)	3.9	dark and light meat, roasted (3½ ounces)	5.1
Corned beef, cooked (3½ ounces)	3.0	light meat only, roasted (3½ ounces)	6.3
Cream of wheat, instant (1 packet)	5.0		
Halibut, raw (3 ounces)	5.0	Swordfish, raw (3 ounces)	8.2

Table A.9. Good Sources of Pantothenic Acid

Food or Beverage	Pantothenic Acid (milligrams)	Food or Beverage	Pantothenic Acid (milligrams)
Acorn squash, baked ($^1/_2$ cup)	0.51	Herring, raw (3 ounces)	0.55
Avocado		Hubbard squash, baked ($^1/_2$ cup)	0.46
California ($^1/_2$ medium)	0.84	Ice cream, vanilla (1 cup)	0.65
Florida ($^1/_2$ medium)	1.47	Ice milk, vanilla (1 cup)	0.66
Beef		Lentils, boiled (1 cup)	1.26
bottom round, braised ($3^1/_2$ ounces)	0.40	Lima beans, boiled (1 cup)	0.79
flank steak, broiled ($3^1/_2$ ounces)	0.44	Mackerel, raw (3 ounces)	0.73
liver, braised ($3^1/_2$ ounces)	4.57	Milk, 1% (1 cup)	0.79
top round, broiled ($3^1/_2$ ounces)	0.48	Mushrooms, raw ($^1/_2$ cup)	0.77
Black beans, boiled (1 cup)	0.42	Navy beans, boiled (1 cup)	0.46
Black-eyed peas, boiled (1 cup)	0.70	Parsnips, boiled ($^1/_2$ cup)	0.46
Buttermilk (1 cup)	0.67	Peanuts (1 ounce)	0.79
Carrot juice, canned (6 ounces)	0.42	Pecans (1 ounce)	0.49
Chicken		Pork	
breast meat, roasted ($^1/_2$ breast)	0.92	loin, roasted ($3^1/_2$ ounces)	0.55
dark and light meat, roasted ($3^1/_2$ ounces)	1.03	shoulder, roasted ($3^1/_2$ ounces)	0.50
leg meat, roasted (1 leg)	1.32	Potato, baked (1 medium)	
liver, simmered ($3^1/_2$ ounces)	5.41	with skin	1.12
thigh meat, roasted (1 thigh)	0.69	without skin	0.87
Corn, boiled ($^1/_2$ cup)	0.72	Salmon, raw (3 ounces)	1.41
Corned beef, cooked ($3^1/_2$ ounces)	0.42	Strawberries (1 cup)	0.51
Cottage cheese, low-fat (1 cup)	0.49	Sweet potato, baked (1 medium)	0.74
Dates, dried (10 dates)	0.65	Tomato juice, canned (6 ounces)	0.46
Egg, boiled (1 large)	0.86	Trout, raw (3 ounces)	1.65
Figs, dried (10 figs)	0.81	Turkey, dark and light meat, roasted ($3^1/_2$ ounces)	0.86
Garbanzo beans, boiled (1 cup)	0.47	Yogurt, low-fat (8 ounces)	1.34
Great Northern beans, boiled (1 cup)	0.47		

Table A.10. Good Sources of Vitamin B$_6$

Food or Beverage	Vitamin B$_6$ (milligrams)	Food or Beverage	Vitamin B$_6$ (milligrams)
Avocado		Lentils, boiled (1 cup)	0.35
California ($^1/_2$ medium)	0.24	Lima beans, boiled (1 cup)	0.30
Florida ($^1/_2$ medium)	0.42	Mackerel (3 ounces, raw)	0.34
Banana (1 medium)	0.66	Miso ($^1/_2$ cup)	0.30
Beef		Navy beans, boiled (1 cup)	0.30
bottom round, braised ($3^1/_2$ ounces)	0.34	Oatmeal, instant (1 packet)	0.74
brisket, braised ($3^1/_2$ ounces)	0.25	Pineapple juice, canned (1 cup)	0.24
flank steak, broiled ($3^1/_2$ ounces)	0.35	Pinto beans, boiled (1 cup)	0.27
liver, braised ($3^1/_2$ ounces)	0.91	Pork	
top round, broiled ($3^1/_2$ ounces)	0.54	loin, roasted ($3^1/_2$ ounces)	0.38
		shoulder, roasted ($3^1/_2$ ounces)	0.33
Carrot juice, canned (6 ounces)	0.40	Potato, baked (1 medium)	
Chicken		with skin	0.70
breast meat, roasted ($^1/_2$ breast)	0.57	without skin	0.47
dark and light meat, roasted ($3^1/_2$ ounces)	0.40	Raisins, golden, seedless ($^2/_3$ cup)	0.32
leg meat, roasted (1 leg)	0.37	Salmon, raw (3 ounces)	0.70
liver, simmered ($3^1/_2$ ounces)	0.58	Sweet potato, baked (1 medium)	0.28
Cream of wheat, instant (1 packet)	0.50	Swordfish, raw (3 ounces)	0.28
Figs, dried (10 figs)	0.42	Tuna, canned in water (3 ounces)	0.32
Haddock, raw (3 ounces)	0.26	Turkey, dark and light meat, roasted ($3^1/_2$ ounces)	0.41
Halibut, raw (3 ounces)	0.29		
Ham, canned ($3^1/_2$ ounces)	0.48	Wheat germ, toasted ($^1/_4$ cup)	0.28
Herring, raw (3 ounces)	0.26		

Table A.11. Good Sources of Vitamin B$_{12}$

Food or Beverage	Vitamin B$_{12}$ (micrograms)	Food or Beverage	Vitamin B$_{12}$ (micrograms)
Beef		ground, lean, baked ($3^1/_2$ ounces)	1.77
bottom round, braised ($3^1/_2$ ounces)	2.40	liver, braised ($3^1/_2$ ounces)	71.00
brisket, braised ($3^1/_2$ ounces)	2.23	top round, broiled ($3^1/_2$ ounces)	2.44
flank steak, braised ($3^1/_2$ ounces)	3.02		

Food or Beverage	Vitamin B$_{12}$ (micrograms)	Food or Beverage	Vitamin B$_{12}$ (micrograms)
Carp, raw (3 ounces)	1.30	Herring, raw (3 ounces)	11.62
Chicken liver, simmered (3$^{1}/_2$ ounces)	19.39	Mackerel, raw (3 ounces)	7.40
		Oysters, raw (6 medium)	16.07
Clams, raw (4 large or 9 small)	42.03	Salmon, raw (3 ounces)	2.70
Corned beef, cooked (3$^{1}/_2$ ounces)	1.63	Sardines, canned in oil (2 sardines)	2.15
Cottage cheese, low-fat (1 cup)	1.43	Scallops (6 large or 14 small, raw)	1.30
Crab, cooked (3 ounces)	6.21	Swordfish (3 ounces)	1.49
Haddock, raw (3 ounces)	1.02	Trout, raw (3 ounces)	6.62
Halibut, raw (3 ounces)	1.01	Yogurt, low-fat (8 ounces)	1.28

Table A.12. Good Sources of Biotin

Food or Beverage	Biotin (micrograms)	Food or Beverage	Biotin (micrograms)
Avocado ($^{1}/_2$ medium)	3.60	Mackerel, fried (3 ounces)	6.80
Beef liver, fried (3 ounces)	45.08	Mushrooms, raw ($^{1}/_2$ cup)	4.20
Black-eyed peas ($^{1}/_3$ cup)	3.86	Oatmeal ($^{1}/_2$ cup)	24.57
Brazil nuts (1 ounce)	3.12	Peanut butter (1 tablespoon)	15.17
Camembert cheese (1 ounce)	2.15	Peanuts (1 ounce)	20.41
Cashews (1 ounce)	3.69	Pork chop, grilled (3 ounces)	1.70
Chicken		Salmon, steamed (3 ounces)	3.40
light or dark meat, roasted (3 ounces)	1.70	Sardines, canned in oil (3 ounces)	4.25
liver, fried (3 ounces)	144.59	Sausage	
Cod, baked (3 ounces)	2.55	beef, fried (3 ounces)	1.70
		pork, fried (3 ounces)	2.55
Egg (1 extra large)	11.52	Tuna, canned in oil (3 ounces)	2.55
Haddock, steamed (3 ounces)	5.10	Turkey, dark meat only, roasted (3 ounces)	1.70
Halibut, steamed (3 ounces)	4.25		
Hazelnuts (1 ounce)	21.55	Walnuts (1 ounce)	5.39
Herring, grilled (3 ounces)	8.51	Wheat germ (1 tablespoon)	1.77
Macadamia nuts (1 ounce)	1.70	Yogurt, low-fat (8 ounces)	6.58

Table A.13. Good Sources of Folic Acid

Food or Beverage	Folic Acid (micrograms)	Food or Beverage	Folic Acid (micrograms)
Artichoke, boiled (1 medium)	54	Great Northern beans, boiled (1 cup)	181
Asparagus, boiled (6 spears)	88	Kidney beans, boiled (1 cup)	229
Avocado California (1/2 medium)	56	Lentils, boiled (1 cup)	358
Florida (1/2 medium)	81	Lima beans, boiled (1 cup)	156
Beef liver, braised (3 1/2 ounces)	217	Navy beans, boiled (1 cup)	255
Beets, boiled (1/2 cup)	45	Oatmeal, instant (1 packet)	150
Black beans, boiled (1 cup)	256	Orange (1 medium)	47
Black-eyed peas, boiled (1 cup)	356	Orange juice, from concentrate (1 cup)	109
Broad beans, boiled (1 cup)	177	Parsley (1/2 cup)	55
Broccoli, boiled (1/2 cup)	54	Parsnips, boiled (1/2 cup)	45
Brussels sprouts, boiled (4 sprouts)	47	Peas, boiled (1/2 cup)	51
Chicken liver, simmered (3 1/2 ounces)	770	Pineapple juice (1 cup)	58
		Spinach, boiled (1/2 cup)	131
Garbanzo beans, boiled (1 cup)	282	Turnip greens, boiled (1/2 cup)	85

Table A.14. Good Sources of Vitamin C

Food or Beverage	Vitamin C (milligrams)	Food or Beverage	Vitamin C (milligrams)
Acerola ($\frac{1}{2}$ cup)	822	Orange (1 medium)	80
Acorn squash, baked (1 cup)	26	Orange juice, from concentrate (1 cup)	97
Broccoli, boiled ($\frac{1}{2}$ cup)	49	Papaya ($\frac{1}{2}$ medium)	94
Brussels sprouts (4 sprouts)	48	Peas, green ($\frac{1}{2}$ cup)	31
Butternut squash, baked (1 cup)	37	Pineapple juice, canned (1 cup)	27
Cantaloupe ($\frac{1}{2}$ cup)	34	Potato, baked (1 medium)	
Cauliflower, boiled ($\frac{1}{2}$ cup)	34	with skin	26
		without skin	20
Cranberry juice cocktail (1 cup)	108	Strawberries ($\frac{1}{2}$ cup)	43
Grapefruit ($\frac{1}{2}$ medium)	47	Sweet pepper, raw ($\frac{1}{2}$ cup)	64
Guava (1 medium)	165	Grapefruit juice, canned (1 cup)	72
Honeydew melon ($\frac{1}{2}$ cup)	46	Sweet potato, baked (1 medium)	28
Kale, boiled ($\frac{1}{2}$ cup)	27	Tangerine (1 medium)	26
Kiwi fruit (1 medium)	75	Tomato (1 medium)	22
Lemon (1 medium)	31	Tomato juice, canned (6 ounces)	33
Mango (1 medium)	57		

Table A.15. Good Sources of Calcium

Food or Beverage	Calcium (milligrams)	Food or Beverage	Calcium (milligrams)
Almonds (1 ounce)	75	Ice milk, vanilla (1 cup)	176
American cheese (1 ounce)	124	Milk, 1% (1 cup)	349
Anchovies (3 ounces, raw)	125	Monterey Jack cheese (1 ounce)	209
Beet greens, boiled ($1/2$ cup)	82	Mozzarella cheese (1 ounce)	147
Blue cheese (1 ounce)	150	Muenster cheese (1 ounce)	203
Broad beans, boiled (1 cup)	62	Navy beans, boiled (1 cup)	128
Buttermilk (1 cup)	285	Oatmeal, instant (1 packet)	170
Camembert cheese (1 ounce)	108	Parmesan cheese, grated (1 tablespoon)	62
Cheddar cheese (1 ounce)	204	Perch, raw (3 ounces)	68
Colby cheese (1 ounce)	194	Provolone cheese (1 ounce)	214
Cottage cheese, low-fat (1 cup)	138	Rhubarb, raw (1 cup)	266
Crab, blue, cooked (3 ounces)	88	Ricotta, part-skim ($1/2$ cup)	337
Feta cheese (1 ounce)	140	Sardines, canned in oil (2 sardines)	92
Figs, dried (10 figs)	269	Sole, raw ($3 1/2$ ounces)	61
Garbanzo beans, boiled (1 cup)	80	Spinach, boiled ($1/2$ cup)	122
Gouda cheese (1 ounce)	198	Swiss cheese (1 ounce)	272
Great Northern beans, boiled (1 cup)	121	Tofu, raw ($1/2$ cup)	130
Gruyere cheese (1 ounce)	283	Turnip greens, boiled ($1/2$ cup)	99
Ice cream, vanilla (1 cup)	176	Yogurt, low-fat (8 ounces)	415

Table A.16. Good Sources of Magnesium

Food or Beverage	Magnesium (milligrams)	Food or Beverage	Magnesium (milligrams)
Almonds (1 ounce)	84	Lima beans, boiled (1 cup)	82
Artichoke, boiled (1 medium)	47	Mackerel, raw (3 ounces)	64
Avocado, Florida (1 medium)	52	Miso ($1/2$ cup)	58
Beet greens, boiled ($1/2$ cup)	49	Navy beans, boiled (1 cup)	107
Black beans, boiled (1 cup)	121	Okra, boiled ($1/2$ cup)	46
Black-eyed peas, boiled (1 cup)	91	Oysters, raw (6 medium)	46
Brazil nuts, dried (1 ounce)	64	Peanuts, dried (1 ounce)	51
Broad beans, boiled (1 cup)	73	Pears, dried (10 halves)	58
Broccoli, boiled ($1/2$ cup)	47	Pinto beans, boiled (1 cup)	95
Cashews (1 ounce)	74	Pistachio nuts (1 ounce)	45
Figs, dried (10 figs)	111	Potato, baked, with skin (1 medium)	55
Garbanzo beans, boiled (1 cup)	78	Pumpkin seeds, dried (1 ounce)	152
Great Northern beans, boiled (1 cup)	88	Scallops, raw (6 large or 14 small)	48
Halibut, raw (3 ounces)	71	Spinach, boiled ($1/2$ cup)	79
Hazelnuts (1 ounce)	81	Sunflower seeds (1 ounce)	100
Kidney beans, boiled (1 cup)	80	Tofu, raw ($1/2$ cup)	127
Lentils, boiled (1 cup)	71	Walnuts, 1 ounce	57

Table A.17. Good Sources of Zinc

Food or Beverage	Zinc (milligrams)	Food or Beverage	Zinc (milligrams)
Anchovies, raw (3 ounces)	1.46	Great Northern beans, boiled (1 cup)	1.55
Beef		Ham, canned (3$\frac{1}{2}$ ounces)	1.66
bottom round, braised (3$\frac{1}{2}$ ounces)	5.13	Ice cream, vanilla (1 cup)	1.41
brisket, braised (3$\frac{1}{2}$ ounces)	5.01	Kidney beans, boiled (1 cup)	1.89
flank steak, broiled (3$\frac{1}{2}$ ounces)	4.71	Lentils, boiled (1 cup)	2.50
ground, lean, braised (3$\frac{1}{2}$ ounces)	5.10	Lima beans, boiled (1 cup)	1.79
liver, braised (3$\frac{1}{2}$ ounces)	6.07	Lobster, cooked (3 ounces)	2.48
top round, braised (3$\frac{1}{2}$ ounces)	5.40	Mussels, raw (3 ounces)	1.36
Black beans, boiled (1 cup)	1.92	Navy beans, boiled (1 cup)	1.93
Black-eyed peas, boiled (1 cup)	2.20	Oatmeal, instant (1 packet)	1.00
Brazil nuts (1 ounce)	1.30	Oysters	
Broad beans, boiled (1 cup)	1.72	Atlantic (6 medium)	76.40
		Pacific (6 medium)	14.13
Buttermilk (1 cup)	1.03	Pecans, dried (1 ounce)	1.55
Carp (3 ounces, raw)	1.26	Pinto beans, boiled (1 cup)	1.85
Cashews (1 ounce)	1.59	Pork	
Chicken		loin, roasted (3$\frac{1}{2}$ ounces)	2.62
breast meat, roasted ($\frac{1}{2}$ breast)	1.00	shoulder, roasted (3$\frac{1}{2}$ ounces)	3.59
dark meat only, roasted (3$\frac{1}{2}$ ounces)	2.49	Pumpkin seeds, dried (1 ounce)	2.12
leg meat, roasted (1 leg)	2.96	Ricotta, part-skim ($\frac{1}{2}$ cup)	1.66
light and dark meat, roasted (3$\frac{1}{2}$ ounces)	1.94	Sunflower seeds, dried (1 ounce)	1.44
light meat, roasted (3$\frac{1}{2}$ ounces)	1.23	Swiss cheese (1 ounce)	1.11
liver, simmered (3$\frac{1}{2}$ ounces)	4.34	Tofu, raw ($\frac{1}{2}$ cup)	1.00
thigh meat, roasted (1 thigh)	1.46	Turkey	
Clams, raw (4 large or 9 small)	1.16	dark meat, roasted (3$\frac{1}{2}$ ounces)	4.16
Corned beef, cooked (3$\frac{1}{2}$ ounces)	4.58	light and dark meat, roasted (3$\frac{1}{2}$ ounces)	2.96
Crab, cooked (3 ounces)	3.58	light meat, roasted (3$\frac{1}{2}$ ounces)	2.04
Frankfurter, beef (1 frank)	1.24	Wheat germ, toasted ($\frac{1}{4}$ cup)	4.73
Gouda cheese (1 ounce)	1.11	Yogurt, low-fat (8 ounces)	2.02

Table A.18. Good Sources of Iron

Food or Beverage	Iron (milligrams)	Food or Beverage	Iron (milligrams)
Almonds, dried (1 ounce)	1.04	Lima beans, boiled (1 cup)	4.50
Anchovies, raw (3 ounces)	2.76	Mackerel, raw (3 ounces)	1.38
Artichoke, boiled (1 medium)	1.62	Mussels, raw (3 ounces)	3.36
Avocado, California ($\frac{1}{2}$ medium)	1.02	Navy beans, boiled (1 cup)	4.51
Bagel (1 bagel)	1.46	Oatmeal, instant (1 packet)	6.32
Beef		Oysters (6 medium)	5.63
bottom round, braised ($3\frac{1}{2}$ ounces)	3.25	Peas, boiled ($\frac{1}{2}$ cup)	1.24
brisket, braised ($3\frac{1}{2}$ ounces)	2.19	Pinto beans, boiled (1 cup)	4.47
flank steak, braised ($3\frac{1}{2}$ ounces)	3.40	Pistachio nuts, dried (1 ounce)	1.92
ground, lean, baked ($3\frac{1}{2}$ ounces)	2.09	Potato, baked, with skin (1 medium)	2.75
liver, braised ($3\frac{1}{2}$ ounces)	6.77	Prune juice (1 cup)	3.03
top round, broiled ($3\frac{1}{2}$ ounces)	2.81	Prunes, dried (10 prunes)	2.08
Black beans, boiled (1 cup)	3.60	Pumpkin seeds, dried (1 ounce)	4.25
Black-eyed peas, boiled (1 cup)	4.29	Raisins, seedless ($\frac{2}{3}$ cup)	1.79
Brazil nuts, dried (1 ounce)	1.00	Rice, cooked (1 cup)	
Broad beans, boiled (1 cup)	2.54	brown	1.00
Carp (3 ounces, raw)	1.05	white, enriched	1.80
Cashews, dried (1 ounce)	1.70	Shrimp (12 large)	2.05
Chicken		Spaghetti, enriched, cooked (1 cup)	2.25
breast meat, roasted ($\frac{1}{2}$ breast)	1.04	Spinach, boiled ($\frac{1}{2}$ cup)	3.21
leg meat, roasted (1 leg)	1.52	Sunflower seeds, dried (1 ounce)	1.92
light and dark meat, roasted ($3\frac{1}{2}$ ounces)	1.26	Tofu ($\frac{1}{2}$ cup)	6.65
liver, simmered ($3\frac{1}{2}$ ounces)	8.47	Tomato juice, canned (6 ounces)	1.06
Clams (4 large or 9 small)	11.88	Tortilla, corn (1 tortilla)	1.42
Corned beef, cooked ($3\frac{1}{2}$ ounces)	1.86	Trout (3 ounces, raw)	1.62
Cream of Wheat, instant (1 packet)	8.10	Tuna, light, canned in water (3 ounces)	2.72
Egg (1 large)	1.04	Turkey	
Figs, dried (10 figs)	4.18	dark meat, roasted ($3\frac{1}{2}$ ounces)	2.27
Garbanzo beans, boiled (1 cup)	4.74	light and dark meat, roasted ($3\frac{1}{2}$ ounces)	1.79
Great Northern beans, boiled (1 cup)	3.77	light meat, roasted ($3\frac{1}{2}$ ounces)	1.41
Kidney beans, boiled (1 cup)	5.20	Wheat germ, toasted ($\frac{1}{4}$ cup)	2.58
Lamb, leg of, roasted (3 ounces)	1.40		
Lentils, boiled (1 cup)	6.59		

Table A.19. Good Sources of Selenium

Food or Beverage	Selenium (micrograms)	Food or Beverage	Selenium (micrograms)
Beef brisket, boiled (3 ounces)	2.55	Haddock, steamed (3 ounces)	25.52
Cashews (1 ounce)	9.64	Ham, canned (3 ounces)	6.80
Cheddar cheese (1 ounce)	3.40	Kidney beans, boiled ($1/3$ cup)	9.44
Chicken		Mushrooms, raw ($1/2$ cup)	3.15
dark meat, roasted (3 ounces)	5.95	Pecans (1 ounce)	3.40
light meat, roasted (3 ounces)	5.10	Pork chop, grilled (3 ounces)	11.91
Cottage cheese, low-fat ($1/4$ cup)	2.26	Salmon, steamed (3 ounces)	18.71
Crab, boiled (3 ounces)	14.46	Walnuts (1 ounce)	5.39
Egg (1 extra large)	3.15	Yogurt, low-fat (8 ounces)	2.27

Appendix B

The Vitamin and Mineral Strategy Planner

The following worksheet will help you design a nutritional supplement program that's suited to your particular needs. First, review the individual vitamin and mineral chapters to get an overall picture of what the various nutrients can do for you. Jot down your Optimal Daily Allowance in the appropriate column in the worksheet, and use the self-tests provided in each chapter to determine the amount of each nutrient that you are taking in through dietary sources. Then, record the amount of each vitamin and mineral that you need to take in through supplements.

Remember, some people may need to take in higher amounts of specific nutrients; there may be factors in your life, such as your personal or family health history, that place you at higher risk for certain diseases and disorders. That's why I've given you suggested ODA ranges for a number of vitamins and minerals. Be sure to take this into account when you determine your personal ODA.

Sample Worksheet	
Nutrient	**ODA**
Vitamin A	1,000 mcg of RE (5,000 IU)
Carotenoids	6–15 mcg
Vitamin D	400 IU
Vitamin E	200–800 IU
Vitamin K	120 mcg
Vitamin B$_1$ (thiamin)	1.5–10 mg
Vitamin B$_2$ (riboflavin)	2–5 mg
Vitamin B$_3$ (niacin)	20 mg
Vitamin B$_5$ (pantothenic acid)	10–100 mg
Vitamin B$_6$ (pyridoxine)	5–25 mg
Vitamin B$_{12}$ (cobalamin)	100–400 mcg
Biotin	30–100 mcg
Folic acid	400–600 mcg
Vitamin C	250–500 mg
Calcium	1,500 mg
Magnesium	500 mg
Zinc	15 mg; 19 mg for breast-feeding women
Iron	10 mg for men/postmenopausal women; 15 mg for menstruating women; 20 mg for women withheavy menstrual periods.
Selenium	200 mcg

Your Personal ODA	Amount Obtained Through Diet	Amount Needed From Supplements

References

GENERAL

Dietary Reference Intakes for Calcium, Phosphorus, Magnesium, Vitamin D, and Fluoride. Washington, DC: National Academy Press, 1997.

Holland, B, Welch, AA, Unwin, ID, et al. *McCance and Widdowson's The Composition of Foods.* 5th ed. Cambridge, United Kingdom: The Royal Society of Chemistry, 1991.

National Research Council. *Recommended Dietary Allowances.* 10th ed. Washington, DC: National Academy Press, 1989.

Pennington, JA. *Bowes and Church's Food Values of Portions Commonly Used.* 15th ed. Philadelphia, PA: J.B. Lippincott Company, 1989.

CHAPTER 5: VITAMIN A

The Alpha-Tocopherol, Beta-Carotene Cancer Prevention Study Group. "The Effect of Vitamin E and Beta-Carotene on the Incidence of Lung Cancer and Other Cancers in Male Smokers." *New England Journal of Medicine* 330 (1994): 1029–1035.

Blot, WJ, Li, JY, Taylor, PR, et al. "Nutrition Intervention Trials in Linxian, China: Supplementation With Specific Vitamin/Mineral Combinations, Cancer Incidence, and Disease-Specific Mortality in the General Population." *Journal of the National Cancer Institute* 85 (1993): 1483–1492.

Comstock, GW, Helzlsouer, KJ, Bush, TL. "Prediagnostic Serum Levels of Carotenoids and Vitamin E as Related to Subsequent Cancer in Washington County, Maryland." *American Journal of Clinical Nutrition* 53 (1991): 260S–264S.

Connett, JE, Kuller, LH, Kjelsberg, MO, et al. "Relationship Between Carotenoids and Cancer. The Multiple Risk Factor Intervention Trial Study." *Cancer* 64 (1989): 126–134.

Eye Disease Case-Control Study Group. "Antioxidant Status and Neovascular Age-Related Macular Degeneration." *Archives of Opthalmology* 111 (1993): 104–109.

Garewal, HS. "Potential Role of Beta-Carotene in Prevention of Oral Cancer." *American Journal of Clinical Nurition* 53 (1991): 294S–297S.

Gaziano, JM, Manson, JE, Branch, LG, et al. "Dietary Beta-Carotene and Decreased Cardiovascular Mortality in an Elderly Cohort." (abstract) *Journal of the American College of Cardiology* 19 (1992): 377.

Gaziao, JM, Manson, JE, Ridker, PM, et al. "Beta-carotene Therapy for Chronic Stable Angina." (abstract) *Circulation* 82 (1990): 201.

Jacques, PF, Chylack, LT. "Epidemiologic Evidence of a Role for the Antioxidant Vitamins and Carotenoids in Cataract Prevention." *American Journal of Clinical Nutrition* 53 (1991): 352S–355S.

Knekt, P, Heliovaara, M, Rissanen, A, et al. "Serum Antioxidant Vitamins and Risk of Cataract." *British Medical Journal* 305 (1992): 1392–1394.

Kenkt, P, Jarvinen, R, Seppanen, R, et al. "Dietary Antioxidants and the Risk of Lung Cancer." *American Journal of Epidemiology* 134 (1991): 471–479.

Manson, JE, Stampfer, MJ, Willett, WC, et al. "A Prospective Study of Antioxidant Vitamins and Incidence of Coronary Heart Disease in Women." (abstract) *Circulation* 84 (1991): 546.

Mayne, ST, Jamerich, DT, Greenwald, P, et al. "Dietary Beta-Carotene and Lung Cancer Risk in US Nonsmokers." *Journal of the National Cancer Institute* 86 (1994): 33–38.

Semba, RD, Graham, NM, Caiaffa, WT, et al. "Increased Mortality Associated With Vitamin A Deficiency During Human Immunodeficiency Virus Type 1 Infection." *Archives of Internal Medicine* 153 (1993): 2149–2154.

Shekelle, RB, Liu, S., Raynor, WJ, et al. "Dietary Vitamin A and Risk of Cancer in the Western Electric Study." *Lancet* 2 (1981): 1185–1190.

Stahelin, HB, Gey, KF, Eicholder, M, et al. "Beta-Carotene and Cancer Prevention: The Basel Study." *American Journal of Clinical Nutrition* 53 (1991): 265S–269S.

Verreault, R, Chu, J, Mandelson, M, et al. "A Case-Control Study of Diet and Invasive Cervical Cancer." *International Journal of Cancer* 43 (1989): 1050–1054.

Wald, NJ, Boreham, J, Hayward, JL, et al. "Plasma Retinol, Beta-Carotene, and Vitamin E levels in Relation to the Future Risk of Breast Cancer." *British Journal of Cancer* 49 (1984): 321–324.

The Zutphen Study. "Dietary Flavonoids, Antioxidant Vitamins, and Incidence of Stroke." *Archives of Interal Medicine* 154 (1996): 637–642.

CHAPTER 6: VITAMIN D

Chapuy, MC, Arlot, ME, Duboeuf, F, et al. "Vitamin D$_3$ and Calcium to Prevent Hip Fractures in Elderly Women." *New England Journal of Medicine* 327 (1992): 1637–1642.

Dawson-Hughes, B, Dallal, GE, Krall, EA, et al. "Effect of Vitamin D Supplementation on Wintertime and Overall Bone Loss in Healthy Postmenopausal Women." *Annals of Internal Medicine* 115 (1991): 505–512.

Lips, P, van Ginkel, FC, Jongen, MJ, et al. "Determinants of Vitamin D Status in Patients with Hip Fracture and in Elderly Control Subjects." *American Journal of Clinical Nutrition* 46 (1987): 1005–1010.

CHAPTER 7: VITAMIN E

The Alzheimer's Disease Cooperative Study. "A Controlled Trial of Selegiline, Alpha-tocopherol, or Both as Treatment for Alzheimer's Disease." *New England Journal of Medicine* 336 (1997): 1216–1222.

Blot, WJ, Li, JY, Taylor, PR, et al. "Nutrition Intervention Trials in Linxian, China: Supplementation With Specific Vitamin/Mineral Combinations, Cancer Incidence, and Disease-Specific Mortality in the General Population." *Journal of the National Cancer Institute* 85 (1993): 1483–1492.

Gridley, G, McLaughlin, JK, Block, G, et al. "Vitamin Supplement Use and Reduced Risk of Oral and Pharyngeal Cancer." *American Journal of Epidemiology* 135 (1992): 1083–1092.

Knekt, P, Aromaa, A, Maatela, J, et al. "Vitamin E and Cancer Prevention." *American Journal of Clinical Nutrition* 53 (1991): 283S–286S.

Knekt, P, Jarvinen, R, Seppanen, R, et al. "Dietary Antioxidants and the Risk of Lung Cancer." *American Journal of Epidemiology* 134 (1991): 471–479.

LeGardeur, BY, Lopez, SA, Johnson, WD. "A Case-Control Study of Serum Vitamins A, E, and C in Lung Cancer Patients." *Nutrition and Cancer* 14 (1990): 133–140.

Menkes, MS, Comstock, GW, Vuilleumier, JP, et al. "Serum Beta-Carotene, Vitamins A and E, Selenium, and the Risk of Lung Cancer." *New England Journal of Medicine* 315 (1986): 1250–1254.

Meydani, SN, Barklund, MP, Liu, S, et al. "Vitamin E Supplementation Enhances Cell-Mediated Immunity in Healthy Elderly Subjects." *American Journal of Clinical Nutrition* 52 (1990): 557–563.

Palan, PR, Mikhail, MS, Basu, J, et al. "Plasma Levels of Antioxidant Beta-Carotene and Alpha-Tocopherol in Uterine Cervix Dysplasias and Cancer." *Nutrition and Cancer* 15 (1991): 13–20.

Rimm, EB, Stampfer, MJ, Ascherio, A, et al. "Vitamin E Consumption and the Risk of Coronary Heart Disease in Men." *New England Journal of Medicine* 328 (1993): 1450–1456.

Stampfer, MJ, Hennekens, CH, Manson, JE, et al. "Vitamin E Consumptioin and the Risk of Coronary Heart Disease in Women." *New England Journal of Medicine* 328 (1993): 1444–1449.

Verreault, R, Chu, J, Mandelson, M, et al. "A Case-Control Study of Diet and Invasive Cervical Cancer." *International Journal of Cancer* 43 (1989): 1050–1054.

Wald, NJ, Boreham, J, Hayward, JL, et al. "Plasma Retinol, Beta-Carotene, and Vitamin E levels in Relation to the Future Risk of Breast Cancer." *British Journal of Cancer* 49 (1984): 321–324.

CHAPTER 11: VITAMIN B_3 (NIACIN)

Coronary Drug Project Research Group. "Clofibrate and Niacin in Coronary Heart Disase." *The Journal of the American Medical Association* 231 (1975): 360–381.

CHAPTER 14: VITAMIN B_{12} (COBALAMIN)

Clarke R, et al. "Folate, Vitamin B_{12}, and Serum Total Homocysteine Levels in Confirmed Alzheimer's Disease." *Archives of Neurology* 55 (1998): 1449–1455.

Homocysteine Lowering Trialists' Collaboration. "Lowering Blood Homocysteine with Folic Acid Based Supplements: Meta-Analysis of Randomised Trials." *British Medical Journal* 316 (1998): 894–898.

Ubbink, JB, Vermakk, WJ, van der Merwe, A, et al. "Vitamin B_{12}, Vitamin B_6, and Folate Nutritional Status in Men with Hyperhomocysteinemia." *American Journal of Clinical Nutrition* 57 (1993): 47–53.

CHAPTER 16: FOLIC ACID

Butterworth, CE, Hatch, KD, Macaluso, M, et al. "Folate Deficiency and Cervical Dysplasia." *Journal of the American Medical Association* 367 (1992): 528–533.

Czeizel, AE. "Prevention of Congential Abnormalities by Periconceptional Multivitamin Supplementation." *British Medical Journal* 306 (1993): 1645–1648.

Czeizel, AE, Dudas, I. "Prevention of the First Occurrence of Neural-Tube Defects by Perioconceptional Vitamin Supplementation." *New England Journal of Medicine* 327 (1992): 1832–1835.

The European Concerted Action Project. "Plasma Homocysteine as a Risk Factor for Vascular Disease." *Journal of the American Medical Association* (1997): 1775–1781.

MRC Vitamin Study Research Group. "Prevention of Neural Tube Defects: Results of the Medical Research Council Vitamin Study." *Lancet* 338 (1991): 131–137.

Selhub, J, Jacques, PF, Wilson, PW, et al. "Vitamin Status and Intake as Primary Determinants of Homocysteinemia in an Elderly Population." *Journal of the American Medical Association* 270 (1993): 2693–2698.

CHAPTER 17: VITAMIN C (ASCORBIC ACID)

Block, G. "Vitamin C and Cancer Prevention: The Epidemiologic Evidence." *American Journal of Clinical Nutrition* 53 (1991): 270S–282S.

Enstrom, JE, Kanim, LE, Klein, MA. "Vitamin C Intake and Mortality Among a Sample of the US Population." *Epidemiology* 3 (1992): 194–202.

Horn-Ross, PL, Morrow, M, Ljung, B. "Diet and the Risk of Salivary Gland Cancer." *American Journal of Epidemiology* 146 (1997): 171–176.

Howe, GR, Hirohata, T, Hislop, TG, et al. "Dietary Factors and Risk of Breast Cancer: Combined Analysis of 12 Case-Control Studies." *Journal of the National Cancer Institute* 82 (1990): 562–569.

Jacques, PF, Chylack, LT. "Epidemiologic Evidence of a Role for the Antioxidant Vitamins and Carotenoids in Cataract Prevention." *American Journal of Clinical Nutrition* 53 (1991): 352S–355S.

Knekt, P, Jarvinen, R, Seppanen, R, et al. "Dietary Antioxidants and the Risk of Lung Cancer." *American Journal of Epidemiology* 134 (1991): 471–479.

McLaughlin, JK, Gridley, G, Block, G, et al. "Dietary Factors in Oral and Pharyngeal Cancer." *Journal of the National Cancer Institute* 80 (1988): 1237–1243.

The NHANES I Epidemiologic Followup Study. "Intake of Vitamins E, C, and A and Risk of Lung Cancer." *American Journal of Epidemiology* 146 (1997): 231–243.

Perrig, WJ, Perrig, P, Stahelin, HB. "The Relation Between Antioxidants and Memory Performance in the Old and Very Old." *Journal of the American Geriatric Society* 45 (1997): 718–724.

Salonen, JT, Salonen, R, Ihanainen, M, et al. "Blood Pressure, Dietary Fats, and Antioxidants." *American Journal of Clinical Nutrition* 48 (1988): 1226–1232.

Verreault, R, Chu, J, Mandelson, M, et al. "A Case-Control Study of Diet and Invasive Cervical Cancer." *International Journal of Cancer* 43 (1989): 1050–1054.

CHAPTER 18: CALCIUM

Belizan, JM, Villar, J, Pineda, O, et al. "Reduction of Blood Pressure with Calcium Supplementation in Young Adults." *Journal of the American Medical Association* 249 (1983): 1161–1165

Chapuy, MC, Arlot, ME, Duboef, F, et al. "Vitamin D_3 and Calcium to Prevent Hip Fractures in Elderly Women." *New England Journal of Medicine* 327 (1992): 1637–1642.

Dawson-Hughes, B, Dallal, GE, Krali, EA, et al. "A Controlled Trial of the Effect of Calcium Supplementation on Bone Density in Postmenopausal Women." *New England Journal of Medicine* 323 (1990): 878–883.

Garland, C, Barrett-Connor, E, Rossof, AH, et al. "Dietary Vitamin D and Calcium and Risk of Colorectal Cancer: A 19-Year Prospective Study in Men." *Lancet* 1 (1985): 307–309.

Grobbee, DE, Hofman, A. "Effect of Calcium Supplementation on Diastolic Blood Pressure in Young People with Mild Hypertension." *Lancet* 2 (1986): 703–707.

Harlan, WR, Hull, AL, Schmouder, RL, et al. "Blood Pressure and Nutrition in Adults: The National Health and Nutrition Examination Survey." *American Journal of Epidemiology* 120 (1984): 17–28.

Johnston, CC, Miller, JZ, Slemenda, CW, et al. "Calcium Supplementation and Increases in Bone Mineral Density in Children." *New England Journal of Medicine* 327 (1992): 82–87.

Lloyd, T, Andon, MB, Rollings, N, et al. "Calcium Supplementation and Bone Mineral Density in Adolescent Girls." *Journal of the American Medical Association* 270 (1993): 841–844.

CHAPTER 19: MAGNESIUM

Ascherio, A, Rimm, EB, Giovannucci, EL, et al. "A Prospective Study of Nutritional Factors and Hypertension Among US Men." *Circulation* 86 (1992): 1475–1484.

Joffres, MR, Reed, DM, Yano, K. "Relationship of Magnesium Intake and Other Dietary Factors to Blood Pressure: The Honolulu Heart Study." *American Journal of Clinical Nutrition* 45 (1987): 469–475.

Lind, L, Lithell, H, Pollare, T, et al. "Blood Pressure Response During Long-Term Treatment With Magnesium Is Dependent on Magnsium Status: A Double-Blind, Placebo-Controlled Study in Essential Hypertension and in Subjects with High-Normal Blood Pressure." *American Journal of Hypertension* (abstract) *Circulation* 74 (1986) supp. 2, 329.

Widman, L, Wester, PO, Stegmayr, BK, et al. "The Dose-Dependent Reduction in Blood Pressure Through Administration of Magnesium: A Double Blind Placebo Controlled Cross-Over Study." *American Journal of Hypertension* 6 (1993): 41–45.

CHAPTER 20: ZINC

Castillo-Duran, C, Heresi, G, Fisberg, M, Uauy, R. "Controlled Trial of Zinc Supplementation During Recovery from Malnutrition: Effects on Growth and Immune Function." *American Journal of Clinical Nutrition* 45 (1987): 602–608.

Duchateau, J, Delespesse, G, Vereecke, P. "Influence of Oral Zinc Supplementation on the Lymphocyte Response to Mitogens of Normal Subjects." *American Journal of Clinical Nutrition* 34 (1981): 88–93.

Duchateau, J, Delepresse, G, Vrijens, R, et al. "Beneficial Effects of Oral Zinc Supplementation on the Immune Response of Old People." *American Journal of Medicine* 70 (1981): 1001–1004.

Mossad, SB, Macknin, ML, Medendorp, S, Mason, P. "Zinc Gluconate Lozenges for Treating the Common Cold." *Annals of Internal Medicine* 125 (1996): 81–88.

CHAPTER 21: IRON

Salonen, JT, Nyyssonen, K, Korpela, H, et al. "High Stored Iron Levels Are Associated With Excess Risk of Myocardial Infarction in Eastern Finnish Men." *Circulation* 86 (1992): 803–811.

Sempos, CT, Looker, AC, Gillum, RF, et al. "Body Iron Stores and the Risk of Coronary Heart Disease." *New England Journal of Medicine* 330 (1994): 1119–1124.

CHAPTER 22: SELENIUM

Beaglehole, R, Jackson, R, Watkinson, J, et al. "Decreased Blood Selenium and Risk of Myocardial Infarction." *International Journal of Epidemiology* 19 (1990): 918–922.

Blot, WJ, Li, JY, Taylor, PR, et al. "Nutrition Intervention Trials in Linxian, China: Supplementation With Specific Vitamin/Mineral Combinations, Cancer Incidence, and Disease-Specific Mortality in the General Population." *Journal of the National Cancer Institute* 85 (1993): 1483–1492.

Clark, LC, et al. "Effects of Selenium Supplementation for Cancer Prevention in Patients With Carcinoma of the Skin." *Journal of the American Medical Association* 276 (1996): 1957–1963.

Hunter, DJ, Morris, JS, Stampfer, MJ, et al. "A Prospective Study of Selenium Status and Breast Cancer Risk." *Journal of the American Medical Association* 264 (1990): 1128–1131.

Moore, JA, Noiva, R, Wells, IC. "Selenium Concentrations in Plasma of Patients with Arteriographically Defined Coronary Atherosclerosis." *Clinical Chemistry* 30 (1984): 1171–1173.

Aslonen, JT, Alfthan, G, Huttunen, JK, et al. "Association Between Serum Selenium and the Risk of Cancer." *American Journal of Epidemiology* 120 (1984): 342–349.

Salonen, JT, Alfthan, G, Pikkarainen, J, et al. "Association Between Cardiovascular Death and Myocardial Infarction and Serum Selenium in a Matched-Pair Longitudinal Study." *Lancet* 2 (1982): 175–179.

Salonen, JT, Salonen, R, Lappetelainen, R, et al. "Risk of Cancer in Relation to Serum Concentrations of Selenium and Vitamins A and E: Matched Case-Control Analysis of Prospective Data." *British Medical Journal* 290 (1985): 417–420.

van der Brandt, PA, Boldbohm, RA, van't Veer, P, et al. "A Prospective Cohort Study on Toenail Selenium Levels and Risk of Gastrointestinal Cancer." *Journal of the National Cancer Institute* 85 (1993): 224–229.

Willett, WE, Polk, BF, Morris, JS, et al. "Prediagnostic Serum Selenium and Risk of Cancer." *Lancet* 2 (1983): 130–134.

CHAPTER 24: BLACK COHOSH

Duker, EM, Kopanski, L, Jarry, H, et al. "Effects of Extracts from Cimicifuga racemosa on Gonadotropin Release in Menopausal Women and Ovariectomized Rats." *Planta Medica* 57 (1991): 420–424.

Lieberman, S. "A Review of the Effectiveness of Cimicifuga racemosa (Black Cohosh) for the Symptoms of Menopause." *Journal of Women's Health* 7 (1998): 525–529.

CHAPTER 25: CRANBERRY

Avorn, J, Monanae, M, Gurwitz, JH, et al. "Reduction of Bacteriuria and Pyuria After Ingestion of Cranberry Juice." *Journal of the American Medical Association* 271 (1994): 751–754.

Gibson, L, Pike, L, Kilbourn, JP. "Effectiveness of Cranberry Juice in Preventing Urinary Tract Infections in Long-Term Care Facility Patients." *Journal of Naturopathic Medicine* 2 (1991): 45–47.

Ofek, I, Goldhar, J, Zafriri, D, et al. "Anti-Escherichia coli Adhesion Activity of Cranberry and Blueberry Juices." *New England Journal of Medicine* 324 (1991): 1599.

Sobota, AE. "Inhibition of Bacterial Adherence by Cranberry Juice: Potential Use for the Treatment of Urinary Tract Infections." *Journal of Urology* 131 (1984): 1013–1016.

CHAPTER 26: ECHINACEA

Awang, DVC, Kindack, DG. "Herbal Medicine: Echinacea." *Canadian Pharmacology Journal* 124 (1991): 512–516.

Melchart, D, Linde, K, et al. "Immunomodulation with Echinacea—A Systematic Review of Controlled Clinical Studies." *Phytomedicine* 1 (1994): 245–254.

Schoeberger, D. "The Influence of Immune-Stimulating Effects of Pressed Juice from Echinacea purpurea on the Course and Severity of Colds." *Forum of Immunology* 8 (1992): 2–12.

CHAPTER 27: EVENING PRIMROSE

Khoo, SK, et al. "Evening Primrose Oil and Treatment of Premenstrual Syndrome." *Medical Journal of Australia* 153 (1990): 189–192.

Sharpe, GL, Farr, PM. "Evening Primrose Oil and Eczema." *Lancet* 25 (199): 1283.

CHAPTER 28: FEVERFEW

Johnson, ES, Kadam, NP, Hylands, DM, et al. "Efficacy of Feverfew as a Prophylactic Treatment of Migraine." *British Medical Journal* 291 (1985): 569–573.

Murphy, JJ, Hepinstall, S, Mitchell, JR. "Randomized, Double-Blind, Placebo-Controlled Trial of Feverfew in Migraine Prevention." *Lancet* 7 (1988): 189–192.

CHAPTER 29: GARLIC

Bordia, A. "Effect of Garlic on Blood Lipids in Patients with Coronary Heart Disease." *American Journal of Clinical Nutrition* 27 (1995): 63–65.

Jain, AK, Vargas, R, Gotzkowsky, S, et al. "Can Garlic Reduce Levels of Serum Lipids? A Controlled Clinical Study." *American Journal of Medicine* 94 (1993): 632–635.

Steiner, M, Khan, AH, Holbert, D, et al. "A Double-Blind Crossover Study in Moderately Hypercholesterolemic Men That Compared the Effect of Aged Garlic Extract and Placebo Administration on Blood Lipids." *American Journal of Clinical Nutrition* 64 (1996): 866–870.

Warshafsky, S, Kamer, RS, Sivak, SL, et al. "Effect of Garlic on Total Serum Cholesterol. A Meta-Analysis." *Annals of Internal Medicine* 119 (1993): 599–605.

CHAPTER 30: GINGER

Awang, DVC. "Ginger." *Canadian Pharmacautical Journal* (1992): 309–311.

Mowrey, DB, Clayson, DE. "Motion Sickness, Ginger and Psychophysics." *Lancet* (1982): 655–657.

Stewart, JJ, Wood, MJ, Wood, CD, et al. "Effects of Ginger on Motion Sickness Susceptibility and Gastric Function." *Pharmacology* 42 (1991): 111–120.

CHAPTER 31: GINKGO BILOBA

Kleijnen, J, Knipschild, P. "Ginkgo Biloba for Cerebral Insufficiency." *British Journal of Clinical Pharmacology* 34 (1992): 352–358.

Le Bars, PL, Katz, MM, Berman, N, et al. "A Placebo-Controlled, Double-Blind, Randomized Trial of an Extract of Ginkgo Biloba for Dementia." *Journal of the American Medical Association* 278 (1997): 1327–1332.

CHAPTER 32: GINSENG

Fulder, SJ, Mohan, K, Gethyn-Smith, B. "A Double-Blind Clinical Trial of Panax Ginseng in Aged Subjects." Proceedings of the 4th International Ginseng Symposium 18 (1984): 215.

CHAPTER 33: GREEN TEA

Imai, K, Nakachi, K. "Cross-Sectional Study of Effects of Drinking Green Tea on Cardiovascular and Liver Diseases." *British Medical Journal* 310 (1995): 693–695.

Jankun, J, Selman, SH, Swiercz, R. "Why Drinking Green Tea Could Prevent Cancer." *Nature* 387 (1997): 561.

Luo, M, Kannar, K, Wahlqvist, ML, et al. "Inhibition of LDL Oxidation by Green Tea Extract." *Lancet* 349 (1997): 360–361.

CHAPTER 34: HAWTHORN

Hamon, NW. "Hawthorns: The Genus Crataegus." *Canadian Pharmaceutical Journal* 121 (1988): 708–709.

Schmidt, U, Kuhn, U, et al. "Efficacy of the Hawthorn (Crataegus) Preparation LI 132 in 78 Patients with Chronic Congestive Heart Failure Defined as NYHA Functional Class II." *Phytomedicine* 1 (1994): 17–24.

CHAPTER 35: HORSE CHESTNUT

Chandler, RF. "Horse Chestnut." *Canadian Pharmacy Journal* (1993): 297.

Diehm, C, Trampish, HJ, Lange S. "Comparison of Leg Compression Stocking and Oral Horse-Chestnut Seed Extract Therapy in Patients with Chronic Venous Insufficiency." *Lancet* 347 (1996): 292–294.

Pittler, MH, Ernst, E. "Horse-Chestnut Seed Extract for Chronic Venous Insufficiency." *Archives of Dermatololgy* 134 (1998): 1356–1360.

CHAPTER 36: KAVA

Bone, K. "Kava: A Safe Herbal Treatment for Anxiety." *British Journal of Phytotherapy* 3 (1994): 145–153.

Volz, HP, Kieser, M. "Kava-Kava Extract WS 1490 Versus Placebo in Anxiety Disorders—a Randomized Placebo-Controlled 25-Week Outpatient Trial." *Pharmacopsychiatry* 30 (1997): 1–5.

CHAPTER 37: MILK THISTLE

Ferenci, R, Dragosics, B, Dittrich, H, et al. "Randomized Controlled Trial of Silymarin Treatment in Patients with Cirrhosis of the Liver." *Journal of Hepatology* 9 (1989): 105–113.

Pares, A, Planas, R, Torres, M, et al. "Effects of Silymarin in Alcoholic Patients with Cirrhosis of the Liver: Results of a Controlled, Double-Blind, Randomized and Multicenter Trial." *Journal of Hepatology* 28 (1998): 615–621.

CHAPTER 38: ST. JOHN'S WORT

Awang, DVC. "St. John's Wort." *Canadian Pharmaceutical Journal* 124 (1991): 33–35.

Harrer, G, Sommer, H. "Treatment of Mild/Moderate Depression with Hypericum." *Phytomedicine* 1 (1994): 3–8.

Linde, K, Ramirez, G, Mulrow, CD, et al. "St. John's Wort for Depression— An Overview and Meta-Analysis of Randomised Clinical Trials." *British Medical Journal* 313 (1996): 253–258.

CHAPTER 39: SAW PALMETTO

Braeckman, J. "The Extract of Serenoa Repens in the Treatment of Benign Prostatic Hyperplasia: A Multicenter Open Study." *Current Therapeutic Research* 55 (1994): 776–785.

Dathe, G, Schmid, H. "Phytotherapy of Benign Prostatic Hyperplastic (BPH) with Extractum Serenoa Repens." *Urologe* 31 (1991): 220–223.

Wilt, TJ, Ishani, A, Stark, G, et al. "Saw Palmetto Extracts for Treatment of Benign Prostatic Hyperplasia: A Systematic Review." *Journal of the American Medical Association* 280 (1998): 1604–1609.

CHAPTER 40: VALERIAN

Leathwood, PD, Chauffard, F, Heck, E, et al. "Aqueous Extract of Valerian Root (Valeriana Officinalis L.) Improves Sleep Quality in Man." *Pharmacology, Biochemistry, and Behavior* 17 (1982): 65–71.

Index